LOVE YOURSELF

Healthy

LOVE YOURSELF

Healthy

7 STEPS TO RELEASE
EMOTIONAL & PHYSICAL POUNDS

STACY SOLIE

NOW
PUBLISHING

1.888.5069-NOW
www.nowscpress.com
@nowscpress

Ordering Information:

Quantity sales. Special discounts are available on quantity purchases by corporations, associations, and others. For details, contact the publisher at the address above.

Orders by U.S. trade bookstores and wholesalers. Please contact: NOW SC Press: Tel: (888) 5069-NOW or visit www. nowscpress.com.

Printed in the United States of America

First Printing, 2018

ISBN: 978-0-9995845-1-4

Disclaimer: The author of this book is a health coach and not a medical professional. The information contained in this book is for educational and informational purposes only, and is made available to you as self-help tools for your own use. It is not intended to be a substitute for professional medical advice, diagnosis or treatment that can be provided by your own Medical Provider, Mental Health Provider, registered dietitian or licensed nutritionist, or member of the clergy. Always consult your doctor for your individual needs.

Dedication

Thank you to my chosen family, my mentors, my tribe, my amazingly strong daughter, my MOFA, my publisher, my editors and most importantly God for stretching me to share my authentic gift with you.

Contents

Chapter One

Set Up for Success

Six years ago, my nine-year-old daughter almost died.

That was my wake-up call. The reminder I needed to make my health a priority—not just for me, but for my daughter, too. That day forever changed my life and I'm here today to help you do the same.

Like many professional women juggling family and career, I was stressed out and struggling to find the time to come up with healthy meals for my family. More often than I'd like to admit, I threw my hands in the air and fueled my life with sugar, caffeine, and "convenient food", then used alcohol to relax and sleep at night. Even though I tried to eat healthy and exercise, I still could not lose those last stubborn pounds. I'm sure you can imagine how frustrating and defeating that was.

I was so busy running a business and being a mom that I not only let my health deteriorate, I never realized my daughter was so ill. She had complained of a stomachache but I didn't take it too seriously. Her doctor said she was constipated and needed to increase her fiber. When I asked the doctor how to do that, she told me to check the ingredients for fiber content. I thought it odd that a doctor would recommend getting her healthy through processed foods, but I trusted the physician and agreed.

We went on a cruise and I remember becoming annoyed when my daughter didn't feel like going on any of the excursions. I thought she was just being a kid and being dramatic about the pain. I had no idea what was about to happen.

When we returned, my daughter went back to school and I received the call every parent dreads. The school nurse called to let me know that my baby girl had fainted during class, was having a hard time seeing, and needed to go to the hospital. I can still remember the panicked feeling in the pit of my stomach. At the hospital, the doctor said there was nothing wrong with her and sent us home with no diagnosis or recommendations. For the next several months I walked around in a confused fog. **I felt overwhelmed and helpless as I watched my daughter suffer in constant pain.** After several hospital visits with doctors poking and prodding, she was finally diagnosed with a toxic gallbladder. Her pain was not due to constipation—she had gallstones. My daughter spent her tenth birthday in the hospital having her gallbladder removed. I sat beside her hospital bed, in a state of shock that this could happen to my little girl.

During this whole health scare, I did the only thing I could—I researched. I wanted to find out why my little girl would get gallstones and healthy ways to heal her. That made me wonder why so many other people I knew were getting sick with various ailments. The one thing I found in common were the toxins and chemicals in our food, and they were making people overweight and sick.

I needed a real solution that didn't feel like another gimmick. After tons of research, trainings, and countless trial and error–– I finally found the tools I needed to be able to help my daughter and myself live a health-supportive lifestyle as a modern, busy woman.

Because of my daughter's illness, I was able to find my passion. That was the beginning of my journey to becoming a holistic health coach. I wanted to learn how to keep our family healthy, while helping other moms to regain their own health and become advocates for their families—the quest became finding healthier alternatives. I was able to teach my daughter how to eat without a gallbladder. She felt better after adding healthier foods into her daily diet and worse when she ate processed foods. So we all started reading food labels and cutting out the chemicals. Small lifestyle changes here and there made all the difference in her health. Along the way, I discovered that I felt better, too. I was so used to feeling poorly that I didn't recognize that I was struggling with my own health. As I shared these tools with my clients, they began to undergo amazing health transformations and organically spread the word to their friends and family.

I went into this area thinking I was going to help people get healthy by helping them avoid the dangers in food. What I realized was the problem went much deeper than that. **Getting healthy for women is about more than what they eat** . . .

It's about what they think and how they feel.

It's about digging into our core, and discovering the blocks we carry when it comes to loving ourselves enough to know that we deserve more. And building healthy habits that align with how we want to feel.

I don't believe there is a perfect diet. I don't believe there is one method. And I don't believe that one way will work for every stage of your life. My vision is that we, as women, let go of the old story of "dieting to be skinny" and embrace a new paradigm of "being and living healthy". Being healthy is about being our own personal best versions—strong, energetic, and empowered, while also loving ourselves and our lives.

This is not your standard cookie-cutter diet book that deprives you of all of your favorite foods and repeats the same ol' "eat more greens and exercise more" advice. It's not about deprivation or restriction. This is about learning to listen to your own unique body and to nourish it optimally. This is about looking deep inside yourself for the things that trigger your choices, and finding ways to make the inner you as healthy as the outside you. This is a lifestyle change that includes body, mind, and soul.

I don't believe in watching the scale, counting calories, or focusing on the physical aspects of losing weight. Instead, I believe in diving deeper to get behind what's been holding you back so that you can achieve real results. This book is full of tips, strategies, and tons of goodies so you can enjoy your healthy lifestyle and never go back to how you felt before.

Most of us already know what we need to be doing to improve our health. Yet, even with the best advice, a lot of women still sabotage themselves and regain the weight. When I ask my clients "What are three things you think you could be doing to improve your health?" I get similar answers each time:

1. Be more active

2. Stop eating _____ or stop drinking _____

3. Eat more vegetables

We intuitively know how to make ourselves well, but not all of us know how to make our inner selves healthy, too. Knowing your obstacles, habits, and patterns will help empower you to overcome!

I have created 7 Steps to release emotional and physical pounds to save my clients time in the kitchen and to lose weight permanently, so they can have the body and lifestyle they want. I will be sharing this very method with you in this book. And if you were to speak with my clients, they would tell you that they feel like they have taken off a coat—their clothes fit better, they feel lighter, and are more confident with what they are putting in their body. **This is about more than just food choices—it's about changing your life in all ways.**

Throughout this process, I encourage you to be honest with yourself and to remember to laugh and be kind to yourself along the way. Within each chapter, there will be a set of action steps that I encourage you to take. By taking these small steps you will set yourself up for success.

Action Step: Read and commit to yourself:

1. Be authentic with yourself.

2. Be committed to your own goals and vision.

3. Be open to experiment with new approaches and practice new behaviors.

4. Take ownership for your progress and accomplishments.

5. Celebrate every small step of the way!

Now, turn the page and take that first step to loving yourself healthy!

Chapter Two
Your Pathway to Lasting Change

"The only thing worse than being blind is having sight with no vision." —Helen Keller.

Before we begin with the 7 Steps to release your emotional and physical pounds, you have to get clear about what you've been doing, where you are right now, and what is your motivation. In this chapter we will lay the groundwork needed and in the next chapter we will start the 7 steps to release emotional and physical pounds. Doing that will set you up for success.

Our lives are often so chaotic and busy that we don't take time to figure those things out. We just know that we don't like where we are and we are sick and tired of the status quo. We're stuck because we don't know how to change or what first step to take. I've created seven steps for you in this chapter that will set you on the right path.

The important part is acknowledging to yourself that what you are doing now is not working and you are willing to try something new. Sometimes, when our brain hears the word "new" it wants to protect us. We emotionally run away and hide or we push ourselves out of our comfort zones and then give up. **I want to challenge you to try a different approach this time.** Look at this book with a curious mind. When we are curious, we effectively trust ourselves without judgement. We are "trying it on", so to speak. Essentially, our brains know this is a trial period and if it doesn't work out, we move on. Tell yourself that a few times—make this paradigm shift in your head. How do you feel? Did you just relax? The more you can get in touch with your body and learn to listen to its clues, the more effective and enjoyable the change will be.

First: Go from Chaos to Clarity

The first step on this journey is *Clarity*. You need to be clear about your goals. Clarity is not something you have or you don't have. It's a skill that can be learned. EVERYONE has the ability to turn their chaos into clarity.

What clarity requires is stillness. **You need to quiet your mind in order to hear what it has to say.** For me, meditation provided the best way to stillness.

The recovering "A student" in me would love to report that I have mastered the skill of quieting my voice and that my life is utter bliss. However, the honest truth is that it hasn't been easy.

The first few weeks after I started meditating were amazing. I experienced increased joy, less stress, miracles in my life, and an overall improvement. Then, like any habit, I started to rationalize cutting back. My life was busy, I didn't have as much time, things were going well … etc.

Sound familiar? I noticed that when I didn't make time for meditating, it impacted other areas of my life—my relationships, my health, and even my bank balance. The perfectionist side of me sometimes tries to take the stage. In the past, I would start judging myself, which made things worse and led me to eventually quitting altogether. Next, I told myself that whatever it was didn't work for me and I just wasn't good at "fill in the blank". Then I'd go on another search for something that "worked", AKA the next shiny object. This was a self-defeating pattern that took me years to recognize and to release. I did this by learning how to refocus my attention on finishing a task and giving myself permission to not be perfect. It isn't easy to master, but it is very liberating.

If you're constantly starting something and finding that you're not following through or you're telling yourself that you're not good enough, here are my three tips to tame your inner perfectionist and reach greater clarity, consistency, and ease:

1. **Get Curious to Find Gratitude:** Turn that self-judgement side of yourself into curiosity about your positive intentions in staying stuck. You might be sitting there, confused. "A positive intention?" Yes, you heard me correctly. A positive intention. You see, there is always a very good reason for the choices you make. I believe that all behavior and experience has a positive intention at its root to keep us safe, protected and loved.

   When I let my perfectionist side take over and undermine whatever I was doing, my positive intention became that I was afraid it wouldn't work, so quitting kept me safe from failure.

   By identifying what you're grateful for, you put your focus and energy on the positive and in this state you can create. One of my favorite quotes is by Melody Beattie: "Gratitude unlocks the fullness of life. It turns what we have into enough, and more. It turns denial into acceptance, chaos to order, confusion to clarity. It can turn a meal into a feast, a house into a home, a stranger into a friend."

2. **Say the word "Change":** Many of us have what doctors like to call a "monkey brain", meaning it skips from thought to thought, never settling down on something constructive. Pair that with the negative chatter that has accumulated over our lives, and our minds get stuck in this endless loop that feeds the negative critic inside you. This is all part of the positive intention—it's your brain's way of protecting you, even though it becomes counter-productive. When you turn those things off, you make room to discover which areas of your life desperately want to be nourished. The next time your inner critic tells you that you can't do it or that it won't work for you, say the word "change" out loud. Then be still and listen. In that quiet space, ask yourself, "Is that really true, that I truly cannot—? Listen for the answers that come from within and take a moment to just "Be".

Dr. Joe Dispenza, one of the scientists featured in the award-winning film *What the BLEEP Do We Know!?*, said that by simply saying the word "change" you are rewiring your belief system and distracting yourself long enough to become mindful of the present state. This will interrupt your monkey brain and eventually, with practice, will diminish and quiet the negative chatter.

I challenge you to give it a try and I dare you not to smile afterward, especially if you are in a public setting.

3. **Take a Leap of Faith:** Start before you're ready and take *action*! This may sound crazy. After all, we were taught that good students learn everything before they take a test or attempt a project. That practice doesn't always serve you well in real life. Clarity comes from engagement and not thought alone. Give yourself permission to not be perfect. Know that it's okay to be a beginner. By starting, even if you are taking baby steps, you will form a habit that will become muscle memory. Eventually you will no longer have to remember to act in this new way. It will have become part of who you are.

Whether you are looking to change your diet, start an exercise routine, change a job, relationship, or perhaps you want to try meditating, start slow and approach everything with curiosity, love, and a beginner's mind. When your monkey brain starts chattering, thank her for keeping you safe, take a step forward, and say the word "CHANGE"!

Action Step: Sit down and define your desires. Take as much time as necessary for this exercise. By pinpointing these, you have a reference point to refer to. Ask yourself: *If I could wave a magic wand*

and really get what I wanted in the next month, three months, or even a year, what would that look like? How would my life look different? What will I—or others—see, fear, or hear when I reach my goal? Imagine how you will feel when you *do* accomplish your goal.

Second: Find Your Emotionally Charged Why

At this point you may or may not have a clear idea of your specific goal or desire. It's okay if you aren't 100 percent clear about exactly how to get there or if your vision is still a bit cloudy. Every step you take in this book will bring you closer to discovering your true motivations, which then gives you the tools you need to make a lifelong change.

The second step on your roadmap to success is setting your Emotionally Charged Why: Why you want to change. If your goal is to lose weight, ask yourself, "Why do I want to lose weight?" It's important to really dig deep here. Your reason for changing must affect you on an emotional level. If you are having difficulty finding an emotionally charged why (ECW), take a moment to visualize what your life might be like five, ten, or even fifteen years down the road if you did nothing to change. What will your daily life be like? Who would be affected? What could or couldn't you do? Would your life be bigger or smaller? If any of these questions caused you to inwardly wince, then that's a sensitive area and part of your why.

Now, close your eyes and picture yourself thirty, sixty, ninety days from now. What is your goal? What would you like to see in your life? What don't you want to see? What do you want your future to look like? Or more importantly, how would you like to FEEL? I'm guessing that you would like to feel amazing.

When we think of reasons for weight loss or healthy eating, most of us focus on our outward appearance. Rarely do we ever attach a *feeling* to that goal. What if what you put in your mouth and the results you achieved with your body were only part of the puzzle? **What if knowing how you actually wanted to *feel* was one of the secrets to attaining a healthy weight?** Hint: It's actually easier than you think. I've found that my clients who have the biggest success achieving their goals and maintaining those goals have a very clear ECW.

Ann—not her real name—was a client of mine. She wanted to lose weight, so I asked her a series of questions to find out her ECW. Her first answer: She wanted to look better in her clothes. Now don't get me wrong, this is a valid reason for change. However, it is not a compelling enough reason to keep her motivated during those times when she didn't feel like doing the work or wanted to quit.

I delved deeper and asked what her life would be like if she was able to look better in her clothes. She said that she would feel more confident and that she would be able to attract a man. At that time, her confidence was low and she believed that she needed to lose weight in order to attract a partner. As we talked more, she admitted she ate whenever she felt lonely or sad. You may think that we had found her ECW, but this was only part of it. I did not challenge her belief at that moment. I merely created a space and helped her create a plan that she could achieve.

After asking several more questions, we discovered that what Ann was really looking for was love. The problem? She was looking for something outside of herself to give her a feeling within. However, in order to experience love from someone else, Ann needed to start loving *herself*. Ann was a single mom who hadn't made herself a priority for a long time. When she spoke about this, tears welled up in her eyes and I knew we had found her ECW.

Your story may or may not be similar to Ann's, but you do have something that is important to you and compelling enough to be your basis for change. I urge you to take time to figure out your ECW. Do not skip this step. Think about it when you are in a quiet moment and can get in touch with your deepest emotions. **The important part is that your desire for change touches you emotionally**

and you know what you want instead. Find that and you will be on your way to success.

Action Step: Take ten minutes to dig deep and ask yourself what having _____ (insert desired change) will do for you and what will your life look like once you have it. Repeat this question until you find out your true ECW.

Third: Set a Specific Measurable Goal

At this point, you have gotten a clear idea about what change you wish to make and why you want to make it.

The third step is to set your intention with a Specific Measurable Goal. Sit back, close your eyes, and visualize what your life would look like when you achieve your goal. Engage all of your senses. When would you like to achieve this goal? Is your timeline realistic? Is this something that you can achieve on your own? How will you know when you have achieved your goal? Take a moment and write down the answers to each question, making sure to detail your goal as specifically as possible. Just saying that you want to lose weight is vague and not measurable. Don't rush this part—it's important to build a strong foundation for your wellness journey.

Now, look at your answers. What emotion will you feel when you achieve your goal? Joy, gratitude, confidence, or contentment? One of them? All of them? If you can tap into those feelings early on, you'll be priming your brain and body to act as if your future goal has already been achieved.

Ann's ECW was that she wanted to love herself. When Ann did her visualization, she imagined herself losing twenty pounds in ninety days and being able to fit into her size ten clothes. Her ECW, however, was about love, so I helped her add in some self-love into her visualization. Her elevated emotions were pride, happiness, and love. From that, we created her goal, outlining concrete steps to get from where she was to where she wanted to be.

Here is Ann's Specific Measurable Goal:

I will take one hour for myself every evening of the workweek to turn off my phone and computer. During this time, I will do something for me: read a book, meditate, take a walk, or play with my daughter. I will take two days out of the week and commit to strengthening my body through a class at the gym.

Take some time to write out your specific measurable goal. Choose no more than two or three actions. Break each down into small steps that are doable and fun. In Ann's case, there wasn't anything about food in her goal statement. That's not to say that her food choices didn't need to change. However, without first addressing the underlying issues she wouldn't have made any progress or achieved her goals.

Action Step: Take ten minutes to write down your Specific Measurable Goal:

_____

_____

_____

_____

_____

_____

Fourth: Clear the Distractions

Even the best laid plans can get derailed, especially if there are roadblocks. Roadblocks are distractions and things in your environment that get in the way of your commitment to reaching your goal. Examples of this could be items in your pantry tempting you to break your diet, clutter in your home distracting you from being active, or a schedule that doesn't have time built into it for working out.

Another thing that can derail us is perfectionism. That was my issue. I told myself I needed more information and more training before I could move forward. If you struggle with the perfectionism demon, I encourage you to give yourself permission to be a "B" student. Allow yourself to be imperfect. In the process, you'll have more fun and be more likely to achieve your goal.

One of my favorite paradigms is: **Progress - Perfection = Desired Result**, and I suggest you adopt this as your own. When we make progress we feel like we are accomplishing things and we feel better. However, when we allow the perfectionism critic to whisper in our ears we can get derailed. Once we let go of this perfectionism, it allows us to step into our desired state and feel successful.

Action Step: Take a couple minutes to ask yourself, "*What's stopping me or slowing me down from reaching my goal right now? Are there any distractions in my schedule or environment that need to be cleared before I can move forward?*"

Fifth: Make Fear your Friend

For most of us, the biggest obstacle that stops us from reaching our goal is fear. Fear of failure, fear of rejection, fear of not being good enough, or fear of embarrassment—the list goes on and on. **If we don't learn to make fear our ally, it will keep us stuck in our comfortably miserable lives.**

There's an acronym for FEAR: False Evidence Appearing Real. The majority of time there is no true threat of immediate physical danger, no threat of the loss of someone or something dear to us, and our past experiences don't have to predict our future reality. It's all false evidence holding us hostage to our fears.

Here are 3 steps to make fear your friend instead of letting it rule your decisions:

1. **Reframe "Should" to "Must":** Is your goal a *should* or a *must*? A *should* will feel like an obligation which will lead to resentment and your motivation will die. A *must* means you can't imagine your life without achieving that goal.

2. **Non-negotiable:** We're all busy. We all have challenges. We all have life experiences that make things difficult. However, we also have the ability to decide what is a priority. What could you let go of in order to achieve this goal? My clients will tell me they don't have time. If you think you don't have time to make yourself a priority, look for the time wastes in your day. How much time do you spend on Facebook, YouTube, Pinterest, or watching TV? If your goal was a *must* then finding that time is non-negotiable.

3. **Makeover Mindset:** Many of us encounter a problem and dwell on the problem instead of finding a solution. Accept the fact you will have both challenges and failures. Things

may not turn out the way you envisioned. However, if you learn from your mistakes and persist, you will be successful.

I had to do these myself. I wrote this book as part of a writing challenge to write thirty thousand words in three weeks. To achieve that goal, I had to commit to writing fifteen hundred words a day. When I first signed up, I had no idea what I was going to write about. I didn't think I had anything original to say. I didn't think anyone would read my book. My biggest obstacle was finding the time.

My mentor encouraged me to write anyway. I had always wanted to write a book but never made it a priority. When I imagined being the only one in our group not accomplishing the challenge and never writing my book, I was able to shift my *should* to a *must*. I committed to waking up two hours earlier for three weeks. I shifted my mindset and told myself that I could do anything for three weeks . . . and I did.

If achieving your goal is an absolute *must*, then nothing else matters. Sacrifices won't even be a question and excuses will go right out the window. You'll do whatever it takes to make it happen. Whatever your goal, no matter how big or small, make fear your friend and commit! You are worth it!

Action Step: Identify any fears stopping you from achieving your desired outcome. Then take your

Specific Measurable Goal through the above three steps and make fear your friend.

Sixth: Set Your Anchor

Often, we get derailed when the going gets tough. We can feel like a boat that is adrift and we can forget why we started and get disconnected from our emotionally charged why. To keep yourself on track, set an anchor, something you can look at or touch that reminds you why you are doing this.

This can be a favorite quote, song, outfit, or a photograph of an upcoming trip. It's important that this anchor be directly linked to your emotionally charged why and your specific measurable goal and that you put it in a location that you see often, such as your refrigerator, desk, or car.

In the example with Ann, she used a photograph of a romantic couple on a beach and her favorite quote so that she could stay anchored to her self-love and her desire for a partner.

Every time you see, touch, or hear your anchor it's a reminder so that you can ask yourself: "Am I making the best choice for myself in this moment? Will this choice get me closer to my goal?"

Action Step: Find your anchor and set it in a prominent place where you can refer back to it often.

Seventh: Commit with a Promise Letter

Knowledge is not necessarily power. We can know everything in the world, but if we are unable to create the habits that move us forward then we will never have lasting change. **Our habits determine our success.** We must identify our desires, let go of anything that is holding us back, and commit to doing it until the new behavior becomes instinctual.

By now you have already:

1. Gone from Chaos to Clarity

2. Found Your Emotionally Charged Why

3. Set a Specific Measurable Goal

4. Cleared your distractions

5. Made Fear your Friend

6. Set Your Anchor

The next and final action step is making a commitment by writing yourself a promise letter. Pull this out on the days when your motivation dips or you feel discouraged. It will help remind you that you have made yourself a loving priority. Then recommit to your goal, allowing yourself to be flexible but not allowing yourself to quit.

The following is an example of a promise letter I have my clients sign. You may use the one below or create one specifically for yourself.

Dearest body of mine,

I promise to:

Trust your intuition

Treat you with respect

Offer you healthy foods and beverages

Love you like you're my best friend

Let go of the addictions that hurt you

Love and appreciate you for what you do

Know and trust that you deserve to be healthy

Allow laughter, play and rest to help you feel good

Exercise regularly and appropriately for my body type

Accept you and be grateful for you just the way you are

Listen to you and nourish all areas of body, mind, and soul

Listen to messages you are sending me when you are hurt or sick

Understand that my unexpressed emotions and thoughts affect you

I Love You

Sincerely

(Your Name)

Action Step: I know it's tempting to skip writing the letter. It might feel silly, but it's necessary to give you motivation when you need it most. I'd like to give you extra incentive to take this action step. Write your Promise letter and email it directly to me (stacy@stacysolie.com). I will then personally respond to your email and serve as your accountability partner. Now get ready to take the next step on loving yourself!

Chapter Three

Step #1 – Change Your Health Story

I'm so tired.

I'm too heavy.

I'm lazy.

I'm not strong enough.

I'm too busy.

These are the sentences that begin to write your health story in your head. We constantly talk to ourselves and most of the time it's not in a positive way. What we don't realize is how that negative talk creates a running tape in our minds that then undermines our goals.

After a while, you will begin to believe these statements as truth and **you become what you believe**. It often starts very early in life. You may have had an experience in your early childhood and, based upon that experience, you made an assumption that you weren't good enough or didn't deserve success. This experience created a feeling which became a mood and then "your story" or identity. But it's more than that—these moments make your body secrete biochemicals you become emotionally addicted to, which is the scientific reason why change is so hard. Even though it is a negative thought cycle, it activates the reward system in the brain. The key is changing what the brain sees as a reward.

Instead of responding to life, you can create the life and experiences you want. By choosing to read this book, you have already made a choice about your life and your wellbeing. That's a fabulous first step that puts you on the road to real and lasting change.

In order to change, you have to let go of the way that you feel about these events and find out why you do what you do. It's essentially releasing what your mind thinks is a lifeline—even though this "lifeline" is doing the exact opposite to saving your goals. This is an area that requires a lot of deep work and is best suited for a consultation. However, I am going to teach you a curated version which is the first step of releasing emotional and physical pounds - Change Your Health Story. This first step has a two-part approach and will assist you in changing your story; and through that, writing a new, happier ending!

Part One: Believe You Are Worth It

Did you know you already hold one of the most powerful tools for changing your health story in your hands? Actually, it's in your mind. By simply changing your thoughts and your self-talk, you can visualize a different reality and start to believe that you are worth this new life.

First, believe this can work. I've seen it work hundreds of times; there's scientific research that backs up the theory that changing internal self-talk changes your external circumstances. Next, shift your *I Am* statements into ones of positive affirmation. **I am are two of the most powerful words, for what you put after them shapes your reality.**

If you are still hesitant or don't believe in the power of *I Am* affirmations, take a look at what Oprah has to say here: https://www.youtube.com/watch?v=6iwnLmh-iPA. To quote her: "Anything is possible, if you choose to believe it!"

The second component to authentically believing in your *I Am* affirmations is to engage your senses and move your body. Simply standing in front of the mirror and reciting the affirmations in a monotone, non-expressive way won't anchor those thoughts in your mind. So move your body, use your facial expressions and actually visualize the *I am* affirmation. If you say *I am energized,* then put energy into it by jumping up and down and acting excited. I know it sounds silly, but it works.

Creating positive *I Am* affirmations is a very simple process but not always an easy one. If you have been on a negative spiral for a while, you may have trouble coming up with a list. That's okay. I have provided a list below of some examples that I use for clients and myself. Give yourself permission to be imperfect yet still proud of yourself. That's what helps you bring out the best version of yourself. As you make a conscious effort to adopt a different way of thinking, the brain circuits that processed your old way of thinking begin to fade.

Here are three easy steps to do *I Am* affirmations:

Step 1. Stand in front of a mirror, look yourself in the eye and say, "I am _____." Repeat this process several times. Note, these statements need to be positive, energized, and uplifting.

Step 2. Grab a piece of paper and pen and repeat step #1 and jot down the *I Am* statements. Read your list of positive *I am* statements out loud. Say them with excitement and enthusiasm. Repeat your list as many times as feels right. It's important that you really *feel* the excitement.

If you just say the words it will not make any difference in your body.

Step 3. Do this exercise one or two times a day and you will notice that your mood improves, your negative self-talk diminishes, and you will start to feel lighter and more energized. With practice, other positive *I am* statements will start to come to you. Add them to your list as you begin to grow.

If you are having trouble coming up with statements, try one of these:

- I am worth it
- I am excited
- I am energized
- I am loved
- I am capable
- I am healthy
- I am positive
- I am successful
- I am blessed
- I am grateful
- I am happy
- I am enough

- I am worthy of receiving

- I am a great time manager

- I am organized

Action Step: Follow the three steps to create and regularly affirm your own I Am statements. As you start to notice your beliefs about yourself changing, and the negative self-talk diminishing, take note and change your statements to reflect this new state of mind. Remember, in order to have a different experience, you need to be different.

Part Two: Value your Words

What you tell yourself internally is one half of the equation. The second half is what you say out loud. The language we use in our everyday conversations can be empowering or disempowering. Those words can give us energy or drain us, as well as the people around us. When you are consciously inspiring others, you also inspire yourself.

As women, we tend to downplay our features and disparage ourselves in front of others. There's a scene in *Mean Girls* where the teenage girls stand in front of the mirror together and point out each other's flaws. It's a behavior we develop when we are young that continues into adulthood. We then pass it on to our daughters, creating a vicious cycle. We must avoid words like "need" and "try," both with yourself and the people around you. If you refer back to the should/must information in Chapter Two, you will see how a small change from a noncommittal word to a strong, definitive-plan word can make an enormous difference. By changing the word *try* to *I'm capable*, or *I'm committed*, you will shift your belief in your outcome. The people around you will also hear the stronger conviction in your words and your tone of voice, and be more likely to support you or maybe even join you on your journey!

Action Step: Start to notice your word choices when you are talking to others or even yourself. Are you using words like: *I need, I'll try, I guess, I suppose,* or *It might work*? Don't judge yourself for using those disempowering words. Simply observe them, and when you hear yourself saying any of those words, shift to more empowering words. Be patient; this will take practice. Over time, it will become a habit and will help you to change your health and life.

Chapter Four

Step #2 - Change Your Mindset with Food

So many of us look at food as the enemy and think it's all about the diet. We blame the food we eat and the diet we choose instead of looking at food from a whole perspective. Meaning where it comes from, what it does to our bodies, and how our choices about food impact us. The Second Step to release emotional and physical pounds is to change your mindset with food. Before we get to that, let's talk about diets, which is where almost everyone starts when they think about losing weight or getting healthier.

There are as many diets out there and diet theories as there are people willing to try them. Everyone is looking for that one secret formula for weight loss. Besides the fact that diets usually deprive you of macronutrients such as carbs, proteins, or fats, why do these diet plans fail? There are several reasons.

Fad diets don't work because usually they are based on strategies for weight loss instead of fat loss. You restrict yourself to a very low-calorie or liquid diet and lose a few pounds right away. The problem is you're actually losing muscle, not fat. When you resume your normal eating habits you gain all the weight back and sometimes more. You're not alone—98% of all dieters gain their original weight back.

So why do we retain body fat and lose muscle? The answer goes back thousands of years to our hunter-gatherer days. Early men and women ate anything and everything they could because they knew it might be weeks before they found another meal. To survive, their bodies stored as much fat as possible. So when we go on a fad diet and restrict calories, our body goes back to those age-old instincts and thinks, "Oh no, I'm not being fed, so I better store the fat; I don't know how long this is going to last."

Another key reason that diets don't last is because we don't address the problem of *why* we are overeating and/or making poor food choices. It's not just what you're eating, it's what's eating you— that's a saying that's been around for a while for a reason. If you're unhappy in other areas like your career, relationships, or have a troubled mind-body-spirit connection, then your relationship with food is never going to be healthy. A great way to look at the whole picture is to look at all the areas of your life: your relationships, your career, your self-care, or even your diet. I've created a simple **Mindset Makeover Handout** found in Appendix A where you can rate the different areas of your life so you can step back and see any imbalances and which area is asking for attention.

In addition, the majority of diets are not balanced and are based on extreme measures. Most of them do not consider your body's unique needs. They are also usually based on a select group of people and since we are all bio-individual, what works for one person could be detrimental to another.

Another reason diets fail is because they concentrate on what you *can't* have. **As soon as you focus on what you can't have, that's all you can think about.**

To truly make lasting changes in your body and your life, don't hop on the fad diet wagon. In the long run, the weight will come back and you won't have developed the tools you need for a lifelong change. Find what is holding you back mentally and you'll have the key that unlocks the new healthy you.

Action Step: Fill out the **Mindset Makeover Handout** and rate the level of satisfaction in all seven areas of your life. Identify any areas where you are depriving yourself or beating yourself up for not following through. Write them down and get curious. Ask yourself if you could let some or all of them go so you can start loving yourself instead.

The Energetics of Food

Have you ever noticed that when someone else cooks for you, the food seems to taste better than if you were to eat the same meal in a restaurant or made at home? There's a reason for that—and it has nothing to do with the ingredients or that the other person is a better cook. It's the *energy* behind the food preparation. When someone cooks a meal at home out of love, the energy within that food is love. Your body will receive and process the food differently than a restaurant meal where the cook is rushed, stressed, and yelling at the line staff. **There is energy in food, created by the person doing the cooking.**

This may seem like a stretch for you to believe, but if you believe the principle that nothing is solid and everything is energy, then you can also apply this to food. Food can be measured in many ways—not only for its nutrition but for the experience it gives you and the energy it creates in your body. So, it stands to reason that the way it was grown and prepared may also impact the way that you feel after eating and even your relationship to life.

You can also use food to change the energy within yourself. If you're feeling unfocused and want to feel more grounded in your life, try eating root vegetables, which grow in the ground and provide heartier, more sustainable energy than a salad. If you're feeling tense and want to relax, try adding in more leafy greens, which grow up and outward toward the sun. These foods are cleansing and provide lighter energy for the body. It's good to choose a balance of hearty and light foods, to maintain a delicate balance of focused, yet flexible energy.

There's also energy in your immediate environment. Eating from your own garden or buying produce from the local farmers' market makes you feel more connected to your home and local community. When you eat seasonal, locally grown produce, the body is more able to maintain balance from the inside out. It is beneficial to take advantage of cooling fruits and lighter greens in the summertime, when they are at their peak in harvest. At the same time, heartier vegetables, such as deeply rooted carrots and squashes, grow more abundantly in the wintertime, and will add to the warmth of the body. It's good to maintain a balance of eating seasonally as well as locally, as much as possible, to stay in harmony with the natural order of things.

The way you cook your food can make a difference in the energy of your meal, too. Cooking on your stovetop is a lot more relaxing and health-supporting to the body than microwaving your food, which destroys much of the nutrients, the molecular structure, destroying much of the food's energy.

Look at all aspects of your food—who cooks it, where it comes from, how it's prepared, and whether it's seasonal and healthy. That energy will translate into enthusiasm for your new way of life and spur you on to even better choices!

Action Step: Observe the environment the next time you go out to eat. Is the restaurant chaotic or calm? Do they offer seasonal foods? How are they preparing the food—over a grill, on a stove, or in a microwave? Do your best to make conscious choices about choosing foods that will give you the highest energy. Remember, this is not about changing everything all at once. By simply taking one small step and being aware, making healthier choices will become much easier.

Make a Food Upgrade

For most of us, it's not realistic to eat one hundred percent clean, organic, non-processed foods for every meal, every day of the week. Sometimes you just want a potato chip or a cookie. Maybe your budget doesn't allow for a full organic grocery list. I recommend getting as close to nature as you can with your food choices by upgrading your food quality. The lower quality foods, while cheaper, typically have a higher chemical count and are processed with more sugars. Cheap proteins also come with issues. In order to stimulate growth and prevent the spread of disease, non-organic cattle and livestock are given growth hormones and antibiotics. Organic animals are not given growth hormones and typically eat healthier diets.

Instead of depriving yourself of potato chips, upgrade the quality from a chemical-filled one to one with very few ingredients that uses real potatoes. When shopping for deli meats look for the ones that say they are nitrate free. As you will see on my **Healthy Shopping Guide**, nitrates are a carcinogen and have been linked to many cancers. Typically, they will put all of the healthier meats together and you will see different brands to choose from. Watch for sales, as price points are becoming more competitive.

Simple food upgrades can make a difference but be careful as food manufacturers use misleading tricks to convince consumers to buy their products and there are a lot of loopholes. With tortillas, for example—something many of us eat often—there are trans fats in many brands. Even if the packaging says no trans-fats, read the label. Partially hydrogenated vegetable oil/hydrogenated oils is trans-fat in another form. Food companies are allowed to put zero trans-fat on the label as long as the amount is less than 0.5 grams per serving. That's why it's vital to read your labels on everything.

Cereals, for instance, claim they are *whole grain* and they are often high in sugar, GMOs (Genetically

Modified Organism) and other artificial ingredients such as food dyes. That's a lot of junk to put in your body.

Don't be fooled by the word *Natural*. Natural and Organic do not mean the same thing. The word natural is not regulated. Any manufacturer can put the word natural on a package. Even if it says *Naturally Sweetened* it can still have processed sugar. Natural is a marketing word, not a truth. Instead, look for the word *Organic*. Only foods that are grown and processed according to USDA standards can be labeled and have the seal of *Organic* on their packaging.

However, just because it says that it is *Organic* doesn't make it healthy. There are plenty of packaged foods that are labeled organic and they are still junk food. The product only needs to have 70% of the ingredients being organic to have the label of *Organic*. So, that means the product could also include up to 30% of non-organic ingredients.

Gluten Free does not mean it is healthy. It just means that it does not have any wheat, spelt, barley or rye. Don't get me wrong there is a place for gluten free products. However, some are better than others. There are many gluten free products that are highly processed, and contain a high amount of sugar, additives, and artificial ingredients.

And when it says *Sugar Free* or *No Sugar*, it is usually replaced with an artificial sweetener such as sucralose, maltodextrin, aspartame, saccharine, etc.

Another thing to watch out for is serving size. When you look at the serving size often times manufacturers will show a single serving size that is unreasonably small to make it look like the sugar, fat, or calories are really low. For example a half of a cookie, or half of a drink are often one serving size. So look at the serving size as this may not represent the entire product.

This may seem overwhelming at first but, a good rule of thumb when you're shopping and looking at food packaging is to remember that the front of the package is designed to entice you and sell the product and the truth can usually be found on the back in the ingredients. And when looking at the ingredients, they are listed by quantity from highest to lowest. Look for products that have whole foods listed as the first three ingredients as this is usually the majority of the product.

Make organic choices with the things that matter most—fruits and vegetables with edible peels, proteins that form the base of your meals, dairy products you ingest—and, as your budget allows, add in other non-processed, organic foods. Fortunately, we live in a time where there are better options and resources are becoming more affordable. Stores like Trader Joe's, Aldi, and online stores have organic options at low prices, and other stores are following suit. Mainstream grocery stores are starting to carry foods that are organic, non-GMO, nitrate-free, etc. You can find these foods and upgrade your food choices, simply by reading labels and shopping around.

A few subtle shifts can make a huge difference in reducing the chemicals you choose to put in your body. We can't avoid them all, but we can be more educated and make better choices for every single meal.

Action Step: The next time you go grocery shopping, choose one item to upgrade. No need to overhaul the entire pantry right away. Start small and be curious about what you are putting in your body.

Look for the Right Nutrients

People often ask me why they need vitamins and supplements, or why eating organic isn't enough to get proper nutrients. The problem is we aren't getting enough high-dense nutrients today. Crops grown decades ago were much richer in vitamins and minerals than the varieties most of us get today because our soil is depleted. The modern agricultural system constantly re-cultivates the land without replenishing the phytonutrients. This leads to nutrient-deficient crops. GMO crops inhibit nutrient absorption. When chemicals such as Roundup and other herbicides and pesticides are used, it further degrades nutrient quality. Sadly, each successive generation of fast-growing, pest-resistant crops is more nutrient deprived than the one before.

Just because fruits and vegetables aren't as healthy as they used to be doesn't mean we should avoid them. Vegetables are extraordinarily rich in nutrients and beneficial phytochemicals. Those things are still there, and vegetables and fruits are our best sources to find them. Organic vegetables and fruits will have more than non-organic. However, we do need supplements to support and increase our nutrients.

As with anything, you need to be aware of the ingredients' source of the nutrients and vitamins you are taking. If the supplement has the description of "natural" on the front it often refers to a synthetic (man-made) vitamin that replicates nature. **So be sure to do your research and know what you are putting into your body**.

I'm not going to cover all of the different vitamins, nor am I going to give you my recommendations. That is an individual choice, depending on many factors in your life. I encourage you to get a blood test to determine any vitamin deficiencies. Talk to your doctor and then research the supplements you're considering— talk them over with your doctor, and always listen to your body. If you are taking something that makes you feel unwell, stop taking it and investigate why.

Keep in mind that you can't add nutrients to a toxic body and expect to get instant results. It's like planting a new garden on soil that is full of rocks and weeds. Change takes time, so be patient and keep doing your research.

Action Step: Get your bloodwork done and then find high-quality vitamins and supplements from a trusted source. See if you notice any difference in your energy. You should start to notice more energy within 30 days. If not, then go back to your doctor and talk with him or her about making substitutions.

Chapter Five

Step #3 - Crowding Out to Have More

Count this, tally that, eat this, not that …

What if there was a far easier approach to eating? One that didn't require a degree in mathematics. There is. It's called *Crowding Out* and it's the third step to release emotional and physical pounds.

The concept of crowding out was first introduced to me during my health coach training at the Institute for Integrative Nutrition. Crowding out is when you add more healthy foods to your meals rather than taking things away. By eating more vegetables, fruits, and other nutrient-dense foods, your cravings for less healthy foods will naturally diminish. There simply isn't room for junk food and unhealthy overeating when you're satisfied and nourished by real food!

It's really simple—start with eating the healthiest foods first. Load your plate with lean proteins, salad, raw/cooked vegetables, and whole grains before you add anything less healthy. You've essentially crowded your plate with healthy options, thus crowding out the space left for the unhealthy foods. By doing this one step you're far less likely to overeat on starches and desserts.

Another way to crowd out is to try new healthy foods. Are you stuck in a food rut? Buying the same things, week after week, at the grocery store? If so, try a new vegetable, a new kind of fish, or a different grain. If you're a little leery of trying new foods, check out some recipes first that include them along with your other favorites. This way, you might find a new food to love. If you're unsure what a new vegetable or fruit will taste like, ask your grocer or local farm stand owner. They're the experts and can tell you the difference and give you preparation suggestions.

As you are doing this, pay attention to which foods give you energy and which ones rob you of energy. Your body will naturally communicate with your brain and give you the feedback you need to make healthy choices. Once you start to recognize the pluses and minuses of certain foods, you will no longer feel deprived. Instead, you will feel empowered because you are in control of choosing the foods that make you feel great.

The best thing about eating this way is that it is customized to *you*. **There is no one-size-fits-all diet.** Discover what works best for you and make that your own, individual plan.

Doing so will help redirect your thinking. Instead of focusing on what you can't have, you're focusing on the foods that have great benefits in all areas of your life. As we discussed earlier, one of the reasons why diets fail is because we deprive ourselves of things we love and focus our attention on what we can't have. Refocus on the great things you can and are eating and you will feel more empowered and less deprived.

Action Step: Try one new food this week and notice if it gives you energy or robs your energy.

Food Prepping That Works With Your Life

For so many, the thought of preparing food for yourself or your family during the week is overwhelming. It seems like just one more thing you have to do—yet another task for which you barely have time.

Ask yourself this: Are you frustrated with your weight-loss because eating take-out and junk food seems easier and less time-consuming than eating healthy?

Let's be real. Life's too short to waste it in the kitchen. It's stressful and takes time to prepare and plan. It's also frustrating to come home from a busy day to an empty fridge and have no idea of what you are going to eat for dinner. So, how can you find the balance to enjoy your life and still eat healthy?

The easiest solution is to have a plan that includes two to three planned meals for the week, making enough to have leftovers. Also, plan for two to three easy meals that you always have on hand, so if you do forget to plan or just simply run out of time, you have a backup plan that is healthier than ordering take-out or pizza.

Here are a few steps to make your meal planning really simple:

1. Select one day out of the week and block out two hours to save you ten hours in your week. Write down two or three meals you know you and/or your family likes. If you don't have that many, go online and search healthy recipes. You can search by ingredients, by occasion, or by prep time. Bookmark your favorite sites to make it easier for upcoming weeks.

    Then create a shopping list. When you are creating your menu and grocery list, be sure to select a variety of protein sources such as organic chicken, wild fish, ground turkey, grass-fed beef, or even a meatless night with rice and beans. Select a variety of your favorite veggies and salad fixings. Choose healthier carbs such as quinoa, brown rice, brown rice pasta, quinoa pasta, or sweet potatoes. Choose a couple fruits and vegetables for healthy snacks.

If meal planning overwhelms you, this is where my meal ideas come in! I have done all the work for you! On my website, you'll find dozens of meal ideas broken down into recipes, shopping lists, and meal prep ideas for each week, based on the servings you need.

2. After you have gone to the grocery store, wash all your produce. This step is *very* important. If you don't wash your produce and you just leave it in the plastic store containers, chances are you will not have time to prepare it; and if it's not easily accessible, it will go bad and be wasted. Also, there are pesticides and cleaning agents applied to fruits and vegetables prior to them landing on grocers' shelves.

3. Get your snacks ready. Cut up the vegetables and put them in glass containers. If you don't have clear glass containers—preferably with lids—I highly recommend replacing your plastic containers with glass.

Not only is glass a healthier option, but you can actually see what is in the containers so chances are better the food won't go to waste. When the containers are stacked in the fridge you can see all the colorful healthy choices right there, convenient and ready to eat. Now, instead of opening your pantry door you can open the refrigerator door for a quick, healthy snack.

4. While prepping your produce, take advantage of this time and multi-task by putting some of your other kitchen gadgets to work. Use your oven to bake up a pan of chicken breasts. Boil a dozen eggs on the stovetop. Dust off your crockpot and rice cooker. Both of these appliances are easy to use. Cook some rice for the week while the chicken is in the oven, and a soup is coming together in the crockpot.

That's it! In less than two hours of prep time, you'll have two side dishes, pre-baked chicken, boiled eggs for snacks or breakfast, as well as all of your fruits and veggies washed and prepped. From this, you can easily make salads and several meals. Try a burrito bowl, a stir-fry with brown rice, or a grilled chicken salad. If you want to see how I food prep for the week, watch this YouTube video: https://www.youtube.com/watch?v=twnvKQTcdbc

Action Step: Pick a day of the week and commit two hours to food prep. Ultimately, this saves you hours of time during the week.

Count Chemicals not Calories

When I talk with my clients, one of their biggest complaints is how much work a diet is, counting calories and weighing your portions. I personally don't believe in counting calories, weighing your food, etc. That's not to say that we shouldn't be mindful of how much food we consume, but counting calories is not sustainable long term. However, reducing the chemicals you ingest is something you can start today and continue doing long into the future.

A hundred years ago, the amount of toxins our great-grandparents ingested *over the course of their lifetime* is the same amount that we ingest *daily*. **The EPA shows that the average American's body now harbors between forty and eighty different commercial chemicals at toxic levels**. As a defensive mechanism, the body stores these chemicals in fat cells throughout our liver, kidneys, thyroid, and adrenal glands. Increased body fat leaches toxins into the bloodstream. The liver then excretes them through the bile duct into the intestines, and through the kidneys in urine. This vicious cycle keeps us in a chronic state of ill health. Unfortunately, we can minimize our toxins but we can't avoid them entirely. They are in breakfast cereals, deli meats, bottled water, soap, the air we breathe, and the clothes we wear. Ultimately, our bodies' defense systems don't recognize the man-made chemicals and can't keep up to eliminate them. Without regular cleansing we have no defense against them.

Our bodies become a wasteland for all of the processed foods, alcohol, sugars, and toxins we consume, often without us even knowing it. These toxins disrupt the pH balance in our bodies, causing pain and inflammation—bloated face and hands, acne, premature aging, painful joints, and the like—digestive issues, and even diseases. Here are the top signs and symptoms of toxicity:

- Sugar cravings

- Low or inconsistent energy

- Bloating or gas

- Caffeine addiction

- Binge eating or drinking

- Mood swings/irritability/anxiety

- Brain fog or difficulty concentrating

- Fluid retention

- Migraines or headaches

If you would like to get more information about ways that you can eliminate toxins in your home

I recommend: *The Healthy Home: Simple Truths to Protect Your Family From Hidden Household Dangers.*

One way to minimize the toxins you ingest is to start reading food labels. Most of us look at the labels and either focus on how many calories are in the product or glance at the carbs and fats. However, as was discussed in **Chapter 4**, the most important information on that label is the ingredients list. This is where manufacturers hide all kinds of chemicals and toxins that make us feel awful, cause inflammation, disease, and weight gain. **We have gotten away from real food and we are eating chemically enhanced food.** If you do need to eat processed food, look at the back of the box—if you see an ingredient you can't pronounce, chances are good you shouldn't be ingesting it. That's what I did with my daughter and her health improved dramatically once we reduced the toxins and chemicals she was ingesting. The same can happen for you.

One common additive we are familiar with is Aspartame. We know it's found in diet sodas and sugar-free products. But did you know that aspartame is also found in toothpaste, chewable vitamins, gum, mints, and cough syrup? Aspartame is a neurotoxin and carcinogen. It is known to erode intelligence and affect short-term memory. It creates an addiction to sweets, which increases your body's demand for things that aren't healthy.

Aspartame is not your friend. There are so many other ingredients you should avoid. To help you, I have developed a **Healthy Shopping Guide**.

The best way to clear your body of many of these chemicals and toxins is to do a detox. There are several steps involved here, but don't be overwhelmed. Pick one or two to undertake each week until you are living a cleaner, healthier life!

Tips for Detoxing

- Avoid skincare products with harmful chemicals such as phthalates

- Use stainless steel, glass, or BPA-free plastics

- Use green cleaning products

- Don't smoke

- Drink lemon water first thing in the morning

- Avoid or minimize processed foods, sugar, and alcohol

- Eat organic foods

- Try intermittent fasting

- Eat high-dense nutrients (crowding out)

Action Step: Copy this link: http://bit.ly/2HSJ0qu to download your free copy of my healthy shopping guide so you can put it in your wallet and be armed with healthy options the next time you are at the grocery store. Start to make small changes for your health, purchase by purchase, choice by choice.

Chapter Six

Step #4 – Reframe Exercise to Movement

When I ask my clients what one thing they could be doing for themselves that they are not doing that would have a *big impact* on their health, they usually answer: exercise. But when I ask them how much exercise they are getting, the answer is very little, if any.

We all know that exercise is good for us. Exercise helps us build muscles, get stronger, and lose weight. Did you also know that **it is scientifically proven that exercise makes us smarter, happier, and more successful** as well as strengthening the immune system? It can also relieve symptoms of depression, anxiety, improve sleep, enhance self-esteem and even improve your sex life.

Yet, even though we know all this, we never seem to have enough time or feel motivated to exercise. Physical activity is one of the hardest things to find time for. With our busy lives, exercising often gets put on the back burner. And often, even when we do have the time, we're so exhausted that we simply don't feel up to exercising. So, if we know that exercise is good for us, that it has numerous health benefits, and it can help us achieve our weight and health goals, why do we avoid it? Or start and then stop? I'm going to propose that one of the reasons is we believe that exercise is unpleasant. It's too hard and it takes too much time. The key is finding what works for and with you, so that, as with healthy food choices, you are focusing on the positive instead of the negative.

If the idea of exercising makes you cringe, I get it. I never thought of myself as a gym rat. I remember forcing myself to go into the gym. I would look at all the equipment and start to feel overwhelmed. It was intimidating. For those of you who love the gym, more power to you. For me, I don't want to have to think about what to do. That's why I gravitate towards group classes, or workout videos. When I hear the word *exercise* I can feel my body reacting with resistance and even a mental *ugh*!

What if we were to reframe the word exercise as *movement*? Shifting from Exercise to adding more movement is the fourth step to release emotional and physical pounds. When you think of the word movement, how does that make you feel? Less intimidated, more like you can do it? Just a little shift can make the difference between taking action or staying at home and sitting on the couch.

When you were younger, you probably moved all the time. You rode your bike, ran around playing games, jumped on trampolines, etc. As kids, we didn't think of this as exercise. We were moving all the time and, in fact, sometimes our parents told us to just sit still. Guess what—now that's all we do. We sit. I recently heard someone refer to this epidemic as a "sitting disease". We sit in our cars, we sit in front of the computer, we sit when we eat, and then we end our day by sitting on the couch watching television. According to juststand.org, we spend half our day sitting. The fourth leading risk factor for global mortality is physical inactivity. More than three million deaths a year can be attributed to physical inactivity. **We are becoming more and more sedentary and our bodies and lifestyle are suffering greatly.**

What if, instead of the grueling workouts we tend to avoid, we got back to doing the things we enjoyed? Perhaps try something new or go back to an old hobby you enjoyed. Is there anything you used to love to do or wanted to try? Jumping rope, biking, dancing, Zumba, Yoga, swimming, playing with your kids, walking, tennis, basketball, or even pole dancing? Try several out and have a great time doing it. Think about the way that you feel after you're moving. Chances are you're a lot happier.

Try to link movement with fun and you will avoid it less.

In the end, movement means making a *choice* to move instead of sit. For example, choose to walk up the steps instead of taking the elevator. Choose to walk to places that are within walking distance. Choose to park away from the store and walk to the entrance. Any of these choices will increase your activity level. Before you know it, these choices become habitual.

By incorporating more movement into your day, you can find pockets of time instead of spending hours in the gym. You can move pretty much anywhere and you can have fun doing it. The important thing is to listen to your body. Instead of forcing yourself to do something you hate, find the things that you love. Remember, in this bio-individual approach to being healthy, we focus on what works for us and our bodies.

I used to force myself to run because I thought it was so cool to see everyone participating in marathons. I wanted to be a part of that group. The problem? I hated to run. I hated it when I was a kid and I still hated it as an adult. I participate in the occasional 5K because I love supporting the causes but I still don't enjoy running. However, I do love how I *feel* after I run. When I'm done, I feel empowered, capable. My mood is always better and I'm grateful that my body could finish the run.

From time to time, I run so I can remind myself that I can do anything.

What I do love doing is going to group classes. The pumping music, energy, and competition within the group inspire me and motivate me to join in. I used to be a dancer, so I love anything with choreography. When I'm in a group class, I can turn off my brain and lose myself in learning the choreography. I like to work out with other people and group classes are perfect for that. One of my best friends hates group classes and gets anxious with all of the other people around her, so she chooses other ways to get more movement into her day.

So, what exercise story are you telling yourself? Do you call yourself lazy and unmotivated? If so, go back to Chapter Three and reread the part about how your words impact your emotional and mental health. Do you tell yourself exercise isn't something you could enjoy? Rewrite that script. Allow yourself the freedom to choose something you have fun doing. How would your life change if you gave yourself permission to just move and do the things you love?

We are conditioned to believe that if we don't do one hour of exercise daily, we have failed. When we can't fit that hour in, we feel defeated and do nothing at all. An all-or-nothing mentality keeps you focused on the negative, which is the exact opposite of what we want in trying to achieve a healthy life.

If you have an exercise that works for you, don't give it up. **Do let that all-or-nothing mentality go and instead make a conscious effort to make movement a non-negotiable part of your day.** Even fifteen minutes a day can make a difference. Different forms of exercise will give you different types of energy. Listen to your body to find the movement that will work best for you. Some days it may be more about feeling ease and comfort, so consider doing a little yoga or taking a walk. Other days you may feel more pent-up and aggressive energy. On those days, choose to lift weights, run, or do a body combat class. The important thing is to listen to your body and create the time. Life is all about creating balance in your thoughts, in your food, and in your movement.

6 Tips to Get Your Body Moving (even when you think you don't have time or can't afford to go to the gym):

1. Something every hour: For every one hour that you sit, get up and walk around your desk/house to stretch out your muscles. Do this four to six times a day to keep your muscles active and prevent cramping.

2. Let's stand: Convert to a standing desk or stand up when you're talking on the phone.

3. Learn the 4-minute Workout: Search for the 4-minute workout on the internet. This is a full-body workout that you can do without any equipment at any time of the day and at any ability level.

4. Lunchtime movement: stand during your lunch hour, use the stairs versus the elevator, or take a nice walk around the office or outside.

5. Shake it off: At the end of the day, when you're feeling tired and like doing nothing, challenge yourself to take a fifteen-minute walk. Involve your pets and/or children. Or put on your favorite music and have a dance party. This will help reset your mood and shake off your workday.

6. Don't be a couch potato: Instead of always watching TV from the couch, use a treadmill, stationary bike, jump on a mini trampoline, or simply walk around while your favorite show is playing.

Use these tips to avoid procrastination and sitting all day. Whatever you choose, appreciate your beautiful body and the miracle of moving it! Even if it is only a few minutes a day, any additional movement is progress and better than being sedentary. Combat the "sitting disease" and you'll be amazed at how energized you feel.

Action Step: Try one of the six tips above to create more movement in your day. Experiment with new activities, and involve friends and family to make it more enjoyable.

Chapter Seven

Step #5 - You are the Missing Piece

You're smart, determined, and resourceful. You can find a solution for pretty much everything, but still you struggle. Why can't Google searches or books help you automatically eat better, get healthier, and feel more confident in your own skin?

Because YOU are the missing piece of this puzzle. Even this book isn't enough to do that, not if you don't bring *you* into the equation.

Step number five to release emotional and physical pounds is: You are the Missing Piece

We've all been there. Armed with information and lists, and good intentions . . .

- You start a diet and then stop after a week because it's too much work or takes too much time.

- You stock up on fresh fruits and veggies, determined to cook and eat at home five days a week and before the week is out, you're resorting to takeout menus while the spoiled broccoli in your fridge mocks your efforts.

- You join a gym or buy a 20-pack yoga class only to find the membership card rotting in your wallet two months later.

Stop for a second and answer this question: **How does it feel to keep breaking promises you made to yourself?**

Ouch.

Your inner critic gets the better of you and you end up riding the self-confidence roller coaster. On the outside, you look like you have it all together, but on the inside . . . not so much.

Good news—you're not alone and you didn't do anything wrong. The current diet and health industry is overloading our already overwhelmed lives with information and bright shiny objects that, instead of helping us create a healthy lifestyle, pile on the stress and add more busywork to our to-do list. When we fail, those clever marketing campaigns make us feel ashamed and guilty—as if we somehow messed up an easy task. Commercial messaging is skewing our perspective and our children's view of what constitutes a healthy life.

None of it matters, if you aren't living the life *you* want. A healthy life is about being healthy inside, in your mind and heart. Then all the other pieces fall into place.

This is about setting yourself up in an empowered position instead of forcing yourself into "do-do-do" mode, which takes away your power and allows outside influences to have too much power. If you're willing to put yourself back on the top of your to-do list, your life and your health will change.

Are you ready to try something so different that it might feel silly? Are you willing to put your judgements aside and give yourself permission to try something so simple that your overthinking brain will tell you that it will never work? I could tell you all day long that it works but the only way you will really know is for you to try it yourself.

Start by believing two things:

1. *You don't have to work hard and spend an unreasonable amount of time and effort to eat healthy in order to stay at your tip-top shape.*

2. *Work smarter, not harder. Streamline your routine and do what truly matters for your health and well-being. Do, in essence, what brings you joy.*

I promise, when you apply these principles you won't have to spend any more time than the average person in the kitchen or on the treadmill.

As I mentioned, *you* are the missing piece. **You are your best health advocate and the only one who lives in your body, so you know what feels and works best for you.** The more you learn to listen to and trust your body, the more you will be guided by its signals. I'm not proposing that there isn't a place for modern medicine or doctors. However, if you are your own health advocate, then you can use the tools and resources to help your body function optimally, alongside your physician.

Action Step: Be open to trying something new, even if it sounds so simple that you think it couldn't possibly work. Start to listen to your body's clues and use that to train your mind. Your mind needs to be exercised to become strong, just like your body.

What Is Not as Important as How

Wait, what? Didn't we spend an entire chapter on what you eat and another on what movement adds to your day? Ah, but there's more to it than that. This is the most radical and effective chapter in this book. Because when I teach my clients *how to eat,* it transforms their health and life even if they don't make any major changes in *what they eat.*

Everyone wants a plan or a magic secret that will change everything, but knowledge does not equal habit change. **Just because you know what to do doesn't mean you will do it.**

Eating healthy food and getting active are only half of the equation. Most mainstream health and diet books say the *only thing* you have to do is change your food and exercise. That's simply not true. You can eat the healthiest food on the planet, you can have the perfect exercise routine and the best self-care, but if you're constantly in a stress response mode it's not going to work.

Let me give you a brief scientific reason how the stress response mode impacts our attempts to be healthier. Imagine a mountain lion is chasing you. You're going to be scared, stressed, and your fight or flight response is instantly activated. When that happens, your heart rate speeds up, blood pressure rises, respiration and breaths quicken, hormones that help provide immediate energy are released, blood flow is routed away from digestion and to the arms and legs so you can run, and the digestive system shuts down. This is our body's way of distributing energy. In this situation, it is very useful.

The problem is, in a stressful situation our bodies don't know the difference between a lion chasing us and a really tough day at work. Our modern day work environments create a constant stress response, one our body doesn't realize is not life-threatening. We've gotten so used to being in a stressed state that we pass off the body's response to holding onto weight as digestive problems or lack of sleep. Instead, what is happening is that the sympathetic nervous system is turning on stress and turning off digestion. So, if you have ever felt like there was a lump in your stomach after you've eaten, that's essentially what it is. Your digestion processes have shut down and are waiting to digest the food until you are no longer stressed. **It is *scientifically* impossible for the body to heal or to lose weight when it is under stress.**

The good news is that there is also a part of your nervous system that turns on digestion. While the sympathetic nervous system turns on the stress response and turns off digestion, the parasympathetic nervous system turns off the stress response and turns on digestion. The key is to get the parasympathetic nervous system working more often.

How do you do that? I'm going to share my **Three Step Mindful Method** that I developed using the techniques I learned through the Health Coach Institute. This helps with digestion issues, reduces fatigue, increases energy, and thus results in attaining your healthy weight.

Step One: Breathe Mindfully

Before you take your first bite, try this deep breathing exercise. This will trick your nervous system into believing you are relaxed. In less than one minute, you can go from an anxious, stressed, rushed state to a more calm state where you rev up your digestion and your metabolism. This is one of the simplest things you can do. Too often, when we are stressed our breathing is shallow, our chests are tight, and we forget to take a deep breath.

Have you ever noticed that when you are feeling anxious and you have a deadline, or your kids are getting on your nerves, you tend to make a loud sigh and exhale? This is your body's way of stopping you and slowing down so you take a deep breath. We need to pay attention to this and embrace it as a means of bringing calm to every day and to every meal.

When I was a child, my parents prayed before each meal. They were so diligent they would even pray at restaurants and I can remember feeling embarrassed. Yet, that moment of prayer gave us a breather before the meal. I'm not suggesting that you need to pray before your meal. That's a personal choice—but I do think it's a good idea to pause, take some deep breaths, and find gratitude. You will feel calmer and your body will release that stress response.

For breathing exercises, there are several options available. I use the 5-5-7 technique. You can see an example on my YouTube channel here: https://youtu.be/LxXrZY1Qa9I If you want to try it at home, follow these simple steps:

Step 1. Take a deep breath and inhale for five seconds.

Step 2. Hold for five seconds.

Step 3. Exhale for seven seconds.

Step 4: Repeat three to ten times until you feel your whole body relax.

Action Step: Commit to doing a breathing exercise daily for the next seven days. Notice how you feel. After doing the exercise and before you take your first bite, ask yourself, "On a scale of one to ten, how stressed am I feeling?" If your answer is above a three, then do the breathing exercise until you are in a more relaxed state. If you're still struggling, find at least one thing you are grateful for and focus on that. Note your experience eating this meal versus previous ones you rushed or skipped altogether. Be mindful of your breath, of your life, and of your meals.

Step Two: Chew Mindfully

The second step is mindful chewing. This basic step is often overlooked in our rush to finish a meal.

There is a scientific reason behind the concept of chewing mindfully. Have you ever eaten a meal and looked down at your empty plate, and realized you don't even remember finishing? Sometimes, even though it was a sufficient amount of food, you don't feel full. This is because your brain was not satisfied with the experience. Our brain is designed to experience pleasure from eating. If it doesn't receive any pleasure it won't turn off the mental receptor to tell your body that it's full. Many of my clients who thought they had an emotional eating disorder were actually not taking the time to be mindful during their meals. By changing this one thing they were able to resolve their emotional eating habits and get on the path to weight loss.

Researchers have said that as much as thirty to forty percent of the body's total digestive response to a meal occurs even before the food enters our stomach. The mere thought of food can trigger a release of chemicals in the body. This is called the cephalic phase digestive response, which triggers us to salivate through the sight, smell, taste, or even thought of food. This means our experience and presence while eating influences our eating behaviors. Have you ever noticed that when you smell or see your favorite meal you are suddenly hungry?

Because of this, you have an increased chance of over eating. So, the more present we are while we're eating, our digestion improves thirty to forty percent.

The brain, however, wants to indulge in the full, sensual pleasure of eating. Interestingly enough, your digestive system and your metabolism work most efficiently when you allow yourself the pleasure.

The more awareness and presence you bring to each meal, the less you need to eat—no matter what the food is. The less awareness and presence you bring to each meal, the more you need to eat to meet the brain's pleasure demand. Mindfully chewing allows you to slow down and be present during the meal. You're then able to experience all your senses as you eat, which in turn signals to your brain when you are satiated.

Here are a few tips on how to chew mindfully. The key is to use all your senses, evoked by environment, sight, smell, touch, and chew.

Environment

- Create an environment that is free of distractions, away from your phone, computer, or TV. Use your favorite china, crystal, or your favorite mug. Make your dining environment special because you deserve it

- You will digest your meal differently when you are eating in a relaxed space versus a stressful space, such as eating while driving

Sight

- Observe the colors of your food and the shapes of the items on your plate. If you're drinking something interesting, swirl the liquid in the glass and note the colors and movement

- Even if you are eating alone, do your best to make yourself feel special with your surroundings and choice of silverware, glassware, and plates. This extra step will feel like you're pampering yourself

Smell

- Bring the food or drink to your nose and inhale as if you've never smelled it before

- Take a moment to enjoy the aromas and ease into the experience of eating your meal

Touch

- What's the texture of your food? Of your utensils? The glass in your hand? Observe and process

Chew

- Chew each bit of food twenty to thirty times. While you do, notice the texture of the food and its taste. Let yourself breathe while chewing. Notice the change in taste while you continue to chew your food.

Action Step: Before each meal, engage your senses using the examples above and observe how you feel. Are you more satisfied at the end of the meal and become full earlier?

Step Three: Eat Mindfully

The third step is to begin to eat mindfully for 20 minutes. This is one of my favorite tips because it doesn't cost any money, twenty minutes isn't that much time, and you don't have to change anything you eat. This step not only helps you to lose weight, it helps you gain energy and potentially resolve digestive issues.

Remember, none of these tips have to be completed perfectly. There may be a part of you that says *this is stupid, this is a waste of time,* or *this is not going to work.* If you allow these kinds of thoughts to derail or stop you, you won't follow through and nothing will work.

Commit to a trial run of this method—seven days. Even if you only do it for one meal a day, you will get the hang of it and later be able to incorporate it into every meal.

To get started, grab a pen or pencil and a notebook or your favorite digital device. Nothing big, just something small you can put in your purse and keep with you at work or while out to eat.

Write the numbers one through seven, one for each day of the week. Then make four columns with the following headings: Time, Feeling, Satiated, Noticed.

On the first day with the first meal, look at the time you start eating and make a mental note or, if you forget like me, write it down or make a note in your phone. Then eat your meal as you normally would. Don't make any changes. I know the good girl side of you wants to impress the teacher, but don't do it. Just eat at your normal pace. This is to establish your baseline. After you finish eating, write down the time it took to eat it in the Time column and fill in the rest of the columns with how you felt while eating, how full you feel now, and anything else you observed about this mealtime. Here is an example:

Day	Time	Feeling	Satiated	Noticed
1	6	Not Sure	Too full	I ate faster than I thought

At your next meal, add five minutes to your baseline time and be sure not to finish eating before that time is up. In the example above the baseline time was six minutes, so the next meal should last eleven. Don't be surprised if this feels like a long time. Observe how you feel. At first you may not know, but as you practice this you will begin to listen to what your body is feeling.

To slow down your eating, put your fork down between bites. Take time to breathe and chew mindfully, too. **Make the meal an experience, not just something to get through.**

Continue adding five minutes to each meal until you reach twenty minutes. Along the way, notice when you start to feel satiated and write down that time. For example, after several days of doing this exercise, you may notice that at around fourteen minutes you feel satiated and at sixteen minutes you feel full. This gives you a new baseline of when to stop eating—around fourteen minutes. Use the extra six minutes to relax, enjoy the environment and aromas for the full twenty minutes. The goal is to find your baseline for when you are full so that you will take the time, not overeat, and keep your body in a relaxed state. Give yourself permission to enjoy the experience. We are so conditioned to eating on the run that you may notice your body resisting. Adopt the new belief that you have plenty of time to eat food without rushing.

Do this for seven days. Filling out the chart takes a couple minutes, at most, but after a few days it will become a habit and you won't need to write it down. You'll be able to mindfully check in with yourself and know how you are feeling, know when you feel satiated, know how to reduce your stress, and understand how not to overeat.

This is a great tool. When you're out to eat, you can still eat anything on the menu. The same goes for eating during the holidays. **There are no excuses except the ones that you hear between your ears.** If you get worried or overwhelmed, take a deep breath and tell yourself you've got this!

When you are practicing all three of these steps, you will notice incredible results, especially if you keep it up after the first week. Within thirty days, you'll have formed an incredibly good habit of being present while eating. This will improve your digestion, increase your metabolism, and create a better overall mood. Chances are, you will also be feeling a lot happier.

I had a client who came to me with poor self-esteem, a history of weight gain, and poor eating habits. She was almost seventy and said she had tried everything to get healthy. At first, she was skeptical of my program, but as time went on and these new methods became habits, she noticed a huge change in her attitude and health. "Stacy, I want to thank you for all you have done for me in the past six months," she wrote in an email. "You have taught me how to eat healthy, not only the type of foods I needed to have in my daily diet, but also how to prepare them. I now enjoy cooking more because it is easier, but most important, tastier. I learned how to prepare meals that were less time consuming, yet still healthy and tasty and my stomach feels happy now when I eat. I have learned how to shop smart through your guidance. I also learned that I don't have to deprive myself of the things I love, and how to choose well when going out to eat. My whole thought process regarding food has changed and you have been the guiding force through this. You have been very beneficial in showing me how to destress, as that was my trigger to eat what I shouldn't. I used food as a means to cheer me up and make me feel better. You also taught me how to think differently regarding certain stressful situations, and to think of happier situations at these times. I could go on and on how you have changed my life through your teachings. I am so glad I met you and feel as though we are more than just teacher, but friends."

That's the kind of success that touches my heart. It reminds me why I work so hard in this industry, and why I chose to help other people improve their lives as my daughter and I did. Testimonials like this make me mindful of my role in my clients' lives and the impact a few changes can have, not only on their present but on their futures.

Being mindful is the key to success in so many areas of life. Start with your meals and then apply mindfulness to time with your family, time at your job, even your commute. You'll find that you carry less stress and that, in and of itself, makes for a healthier and happier life.

This mindfulness method is all about connecting with our bodies and relearning how to listen to what we truly crave. When we don't slow down we are disconnected from the messages that our bodies send us.

Action Step: Commit to following these three steps: practice breathing, chewing, and eating mindfully at every meal for one week and write down your observations about how it changes your dining experience. See Addendum B for an example of the Eating Mindfully Chart. Notice your waistline getting smaller and your enjoyment of life getting larger.

Chapter Eight

Step #6 – Deconstructing Your Cravings

You had a bad day, received unwanted news, or you sat home alone on a Friday night—whatever the reason, emotional eating is a reality for many of us. There are many different emotional states that can trigger us to eat for comfort: Stress, anxiety, loneliness, depression, boredom, or even celebrations. Most people have one of those categories that is their main trigger for overeating. Recognizing your emotional trigger and deconstructing your cravings is the sixth step towards release emotional and physical pounds.

Our bodies talk to us all the time. Those messages can have a negative or positive impact—it's up to you. Ultimately, our bodies love us and are constantly busy doing everything they can to keep us alive and functioning. However, **a body can only work with what it's given.**

If you feed it junk, overeat, deprive it of sleep, drink too much alcohol, or ingest too many toxins, your body *will* keep on running. If you crave carbs or sugar when you're having a bad day and indulge, your body *will* keep moving—but not at its best. Like a car, a body can only work with the fuel it's given; give it inferior fuel and you will see inferior results. Start to understand your cravings so you can start building a loving relationship with your own body.

Why Do You Crave That Food?

Have you ever come home from a hectic day at the office and found yourself staring at the pantry? You reach in and grab the chips, crackers, cookies, or something to shove in your mouth because you feel so hungry. Yet no matter how much you eat, you don't feel satisfied. Sometimes this is because you're not physically hungry but rather *soulfully* hungry.

Our bodies have many types of cravings. Food cravings for things like sugar and carbs often come about because we are ignoring other areas of our lives, especially our emotional lives.

Many people view cravings as weakness, but acknowledging them and knowing where they are coming from is very important. **Cravings are our body's way of sending a message about maintaining balance.** When we tune into our bodies and truly listen, we can find out what part of our life needs attention and uncover the keys to your relationship between your body, the food you eat, and your level of health.

I don't believe that cravings are due to lack of willpower or discipline. Remember in the second chapter how we talked about positive intention? Even "bad" behaviors have positive intentions at their core. The best way to deconstruct your cravings is to approach them with curiosity versus judgement. If you judge yourself and beat yourself up for the craving, or for acting on it by overeating, you will never find out why you are doing what you are doing. Therefore, you will never be able to change. However, if you approach your craving— or any behavior you're unhappy with—with curiosity, you can love yourself even if you don't like the behavior. This will help you to separate yourself from the behavior so you reach the true underlying cause.

Deconstructing Your Craving

When you experience a craving, look at not only the food you're reaching for, but also the lifestyle influences of that choice. Ask yourself, "What does my body truly want? Am I getting enough love in my life? How happy am I with my relationships and my work? Do I give myself any downtime or self-care?" The key to stopping a craving is to understand what your body and mind are truly craving.

If you are unhappy with areas of your life and you ignore those signs, your body will instinctually slow you down and signal cravings to nourish you. Just as your body knows how to breathe and pump your heart, your body knows that you require sleep, relaxation, activity, and time for fun.

Of all the relationships in our life, the one with our body is the most essential. Your body craves communication, love, and nurturing. As we discussed in the last chapter, our brains crave pleasure. So, if we deny ourselves the pleasure of eating mindfully, we might also trigger cravings. Even if we indulge in the cravings, we will still feel unfulfilled.

As you learn to deconstruct and respond to your body's cravings, you will create a deep and lasting level of health and balance. You will begin to feel at ease with your choices and you will tune inward versus outward and trust your own intuition. That's when true change can happen.

Here are five easy steps you can take to easily deconstruct your craving and decide if it is a good choice for you:

1. Close your eyes and take a deep breath and ask yourself: *What is it that I'm really craving*? Are you living a life that is

too stressful and your body needs some relaxation and love? Or perhaps you are bored and you need to add some fun in your life? Or is it that actual experience or taste of the food?

2. Have a glass of water and step into the feeling that you would experience if you indulged in that craving. Move past just the taste and move into how you would *feel*.

3. On a scale of one to ten, with one being *Feels Awful* and ten *Feels Awesome,* rate the following questions:

   • How will this make me feel physically? Will my body feel more energized or tired?

   • How will this make me feel emotionally? Will I feel guilty or irritable?

   • How will it make me feel mentally? Will I regret it or feel healthful?

   Rate each one and then average the three questions. If you rated an average of five or more, allow yourself the choice and move on to the fifth step. Note you are making a choice and not falling victim to the craving. If it is below 5 then it is not a nurturing choice and move on to the fourth step.

4. Wait ten minutes, and if you still have a strong craving choose a healthier option.

For example, if you're craving something sweet like chocolate cake, eat some berries, an apple with nut butter, a date, or even a piece of dark chocolate.

5. If after all of that, you still want to indulge in your cravings, then do so and be sure to savor the food. Using the mindful method discussed in the last chapter, engage your senses to smell, taste, and enjoy the food. Don't feel guilty; instead notice the effects on your body. How is this food making you *feel*? Now you can be more aware and free to decide if you really want to eat that next time.

Action Step: The next time you have a craving, treat it as a loving message from your body without judgement. Then get curious and follow the five steps above to assess and deconstruct it.

Emotional Fitness

Most people come to see me because they want to feel better. They either want to move away from a negative feeling or they want to feel happy, at peace, and better in their body.

Have you ever noticed that when you feel joyful, energetic, and are in a great mood that life seems easier and you want to make healthy choices? On the other hand, when you are in a bad mood, a slump, or just don't feel joyful, are you less motivated, feel stuck, and fall off track with your health goals?

So, an important aspect of staying healthy and committed is to keep your emotions healthy as well. What if I told you that you didn't need an excuse to feel good and that energy is a choice? That you can build your emotional fitness, just as you build your physical fitness?

When you feel your energy is low and you want to stay motivated but just don't *feel* like it, I suggest you take a moment to change your emotional fitness. It's just as vital as anything else you do to make yourself stronger and healthier.

How does it work? Well, there's a phrase: **"Emotion is created through motion."** If your emotional state is low or you're in a bad mood, you're not going to feel like being physically active. This compounds on itself—the less you work out, the more impact that has on your emotions and can create a downward spiral of neglecting your health.

Motion and movement are good for more than just raising your heart rate. How you move your body changes your biochemistry. It can change your mood, as well as change the way you experience events in life. Basically, the way you feel emotionally affects the way you feel physically and vice versa.

We need more energy to have more joy in our life. So when we are in a joyful state, our emotional fitness will build, causing a ripple effect for the rest of our health.

If you are in a bad mood and you want to change your emotional state, move your body. It sounds simplistic, but it works. Have you ever done some form of activity and at the end you felt an adrenaline rush and just felt good in your body? What was your mood like? Were you happy or sad? Chances are you felt alive and energized, and ready to tackle anything that came your way. Keep in mind that this form of motion does not need to be a workout or anything that takes a great length of time. All you need to do is change whatever you are doing. So, if you are sitting, stand up and move around. If you are in a noisy room, find a quiet spot. Or if it's quiet, put some music on and dance around.

Here are a few simple ways to keep emotionally fit so you can feel better and stay on track with your health goals:

1. Change your posture: If you notice that your shoulders are hunched, your eyes are cast downward, or your breathing is shallow, then stand upright, set your shoulders back and tilt your head up. Take a couple of deep, long, loving breaths. This slight shift in your posture can increase your confidence and boost your mood.

2. Smile: Change your facial expression to a smile. By simply smiling you will improve your mood.

3. Laugh: Watch your favorite comedian or a silly video on YouTube. Even if you don't feel like changing, you will naturally feel better by simply laughing.

Action Step: The next time you don't feel like doing anything healthy or being active, use one of the above Emotional Fitness tips to change your mood. If those don't resonate, create a few personal ones for yourself that will immediately uplift your mood. Sometimes, just changing your environment for a few minutes is all it takes to hit the reset button. Remember, you may not be able to control your experiences in life but you do have a choice about how you want to feel and be.

Chapter Nine
Step #7 – Self-Nourishment

Somewhere along the way we got lost. We had kids, and our dreams and desires got put on the backburner. Eventually we ended up feeling lost, unappreciated, and even resentful. Then we felt guilty for having those feelings because we "have it all". Aren't we supposed to be grateful and content? If we are going to take back our health we need to look at things differently.

Self-care is a word that can often make people cringe. We know we're supposed to do it, because it's crucial we take care of ourselves. At the same time, we don't want to be selfish and we often feel guilty if we take time for ourselves because that means we are taking time away from our family or career. So how can we possibly fit it all in? The answer is we can't. We have to make some adjustments and prioritize things. The key here is to give your life some peace by being wise about your self-care. **When we take control of our days versus letting**

our days control us, we replenish our physical, mental, and emotional well-being—and that is self-care at its best.

When you hear the word self-nourishment, does that evoke different feelings than the word self-care? To me, the word self-care has been overused and has become associated with the word selfish. What if we reframed it to self-nourishment? To survive, our bodies need food for nourishment and so do our mind and our spirit. Nourishment is something our bodies naturally crave on a physical, mental, and spiritual level and it is the seventh and final step to release emotional and physical pounds. You can look at self-nourishment as just one more piece in that puzzle.

So, where do you start? With doing things you enjoy because that creates happiness. You don't have to spend a lot of money or do something extravagant. You can start with something as simple as taking a walk, spending quiet time with someone you love, listening to music, or reading for fun.

This is not being selfish. This is putting yourself first, which is the same basic concept we talked about earlier in the book—if you don't put the oxygen mask on yourself, you won't be strong enough or capable enough of taking care of the people around you. The paradox is simple—if you make your self-nourishment a priority, you have more to give. You are replenishing your soul and heart, and that in turn creates more of both.

If you have followed along with the tips in this book and already completed some of the action steps by setting goals, changing some eating habits, being more mindful, etc., then you have already taken a huge step in giving yourself more self-nourishment. In time, this investment will pay off over and over again. It's refilling the well from the deepest recesses of yourself, which will only create an even more positive and healthy base for your future.

Action Step: Take a look at your typical day. Where are you giving your time away? Where are you spending your time on things that sap your energy versus filling you up? Find five, ten, even fifteen minutes and schedule time to nourish yourself. I promise that if you make time for yourself you will be more productive with your time, with your family, and your career. You will feel more energized and you won't feel drained when you are hit by setbacks or challenging days.

Celebrate and Compliment Yourself

When you reflect over the past few weeks, have you taken some of the action steps? Have you made any progress? I bet that your first answer was *no, I haven't done all of them*, or *I haven't done them as well as I should*, or *my progress is slower than I want*.

Even if you have done some but not all, the chances are good that you are beating yourself up for falling short in one area or another. We are our own worst critics and we tend to overlook or minimize our accomplishments. It's as if we are waiting for the big win, the giant trophy, or a seal of approval, before we can let loose and celebrate. I look around at all of the amazing women in my life: friends, clients, and mentors. Too many of them tend to diminish their accomplishments. We disparage ourselves or brush off compliments we receive, instead of taking the compliment as the gift it was meant to be.

In the last few days, has someone given you a compliment? What did they say? How did you respond? Or even better, did you do something in the last twenty-four hours that deserved a compliment or a congratulatory pat on the back? How did you respond to yourself? Did you diminish it? Or did you celebrate and tell yourself "Good job!" If your best friend had accomplished the same feat, you would have congratulated her or told her how proud you were. **Treat yourself as if you are your best friend**. Celebrate and compliment yourself on a regular basis.

As you start to make changes in your life, people are going to notice—and some of those people are going to give you a compliment. If you're not prepared to receive the compliment and step into this new version of yourself, you're going to diminish your progress. Before you know it, you will give up on your new goal. Why? Because it's more comfortable to fall back into old bad patterns than to change to new ones. Your brain wants to keep you safe and your body is comfortable with the old ways . . . remember Chapter Three!

In order to prepare yourself for the changes you are making and to calm your brain, you need to learn to celebrate every milestone along the way. When you tell yourself *good job*, or you do something to celebrate, your brain will associate that change with a pleasurable experience. On the flip side, if you berate yourself or criticize yourself for only losing five pounds or eating that slice of cake, then guess what? You will begin to associate these new changes with a negative experience and your motivation will drop even more.

This all makes sense on a conscious level, but that still doesn't mean we'll apply it. Look at this from another angle. If your daughter wanted something and you told her she had to save her money in order to buy it, she may not get that excited. Any long-term plan is hard to celebrate and, like the rest of us, she wants instant gratification by receiving the item right away. However, if you made the savings process fun for her along the way by celebrating her successes and telling her how proud you are every time she saved or worked to earn money, how do you think she would feel? How would that experience be different for her if you shamed her for not saving enough, berated her for not working hard enough, or constantly told her she would never reach her goal? Do you think she might give up? Do you think she would be motivated to save? When we take a step back and see how we are treating ourselves versus how we treat others, we can see that it is no wonder that we give up on ourselves or get frustrated and don't have any fun. **If you change your perspective you can change your results.**

Look at yourself as your own personal coach or sports team fan. When you start to get down on yourself and you don't feel like taking that next step, give yourself a pep talk. Instead of focusing on the negatives or shortcomings, think instead about the progress you have made and celebrate like your favorite team has won a championship.

Action Step: Start to notice when you're talking critically about yourself and shift those words into a compliment. You deserve to experience pleasure and to take pride in your accomplishments. Take a moment to write down a list of things that make you feel good: a hot bath, a long walk, a manicure, etc. We want this to be a menu that you can choose from and celebrate your success.

Here are a few examples of a self-nourishment menu. Use some of these or create your own:

1. Jump up and down and scream, "Yes! I did it!"

2. Put on your favorite song and dance like no one is watching

3. Go outside barefoot. Close your eyes and let the warm sun energize you and fill your heart with gratitude

4. Take a bath with Epsom salts and candles

5. Take yourself out on a movie date

6. Read a book just for fun

7. Color a page or draw a picture with fun markers

8. Watch a really funny movie and laugh hard

9. Go to a play

10. Do a craft

11. Get a facial

12. Get a massage

13. Call a friend you have missed

14. Make a date with one of your children

15. Go out to lunch with your best friend

Love Your Body

I spent the majority of my life hating my body. In elementary school, I was so skinny that I would get made fun of. Then when I hit puberty, I noticed my thighs were getting bigger and began rubbing together. Everything was changing, and even when I exercised more or deprived myself of food I still didn't feel satisfied. Everywhere I looked there were images of beautiful women that were everything that I felt I wasn't. As I look back at that little girl, I wish I could show her how beautiful and special she was and that there was no shame in her body.

Unfortunately, there is so much body shame with little girls and women. Most of my clients struggle with body shame and being able to love themselves. They often say that they want to lose weight or get into shape so they can be happy with themselves and feel better. However, my belief is that **in order to lose the weight or get healthier you must learn to love yourself first.**

Have you ever walked by the mirror in the morning and thought, *ugh I look terrible. My skin looks tired. Look at those wrinkles. Where did that pimple come from*?

Those behaviors undermine your ability to love yourself. We have to learn to love ourselves with total acceptance. To be fine with who we are, just the way we are. Then are in a state of compassion and we are able to make conscious and subconscious choices that will nourish instead of harm ourselves. Authentically loving yourself requires giving yourself attention, acceptance, and appreciation. Doing this will help silence your inner critic and replace negative thoughts with kinder, more loving ones.

Loving yourself is not something that happens overnight. It didn't for me and it probably won't for you. Most of my clients feel like it is an impossible task. This is something that takes time and practice. When you align yourself with the belief that you can do anything and you just need to break it down into chunks, it doesn't feel insurmountable.

The first step is to identify the behavior you want to change and approach it with curiosity versus judgement. Because if you are already judging yourself and you ask yourself questions like *why do I do this* or *how come I do that*, you are judging and not questioning your choices and you feel overwhelmed, sending yourself right back down the rabbit hole. However, when you switch to curiosity instead of asking *why* or *how* questions, you release the judgement.

Curiosity sounds like: *Hmm, that's interesting . . . I wonder what is going on.* Then you can step back and look at it through a new lens and ask yourself if that belief is really your truth or perhaps the echoes of past experiences.

This doesn't mean that everything will be rosy and you won't have any difficulties. In fact, as you practice some of these techniques you might feel like things are getting more difficult. These challenges are a sign that you are growing and changing. Keep at it, and eventually this will become second nature.

Next, in order to feel like you have love and belonging **you have to *believe* that you're worthy of love and belonging.** Logically, this makes sense. However, for many women it's not really that simple. You have to give yourself permission to be yourself and be compassionate when you're not perfect. You have to be willing to let go of who you think you should be in order to be who you authentically are—if that makes sense. Be yourself, without apology; and when you are feeling down or weak, be willing to ask for help because being vulnerable is being a hundred percent authentic.

One of my favorite quotes by Ralph Waldo Emerson is: *Be yourself; no base imitator of another, but your best self. There is something which you can do better than another. Listen to the inward voice and bravely obey that. Do the things at which you are great, not what you were never made for.*

When you notice the wrinkles on your face, appreciate the smile lines and remember those moments that made you smile. If you see dimples on your thighs be grateful for allowing your body to be strong enough to walk and move. The more that we can be grateful for our body's capabilities and beauty, the more we will be able to release the guilt and shame holding us back from being our healthiest.

If you believe your body has the capability to heal itself given the right environment, then you should also believe that this applies to self-love and your inner image of yourself. **When we love our present state, we reduce our stress and anxiety.** In response, our bodies will naturally crave things that are more healthy and loving.

Action Step: The next time you walk by a mirror, find one thing about yourself for which you are grateful and feel love for that part of you. It might be your hair, the color of your eyes, or the dimple in your cheek.

Maintain a Sense of Gratitude

We've talked a lot about being grateful—for your body, for your ability to move, for your life. It's easy to write about gratitude, easy to read about it, but putting it into regular practice can be difficult. It's worth making gratitude a key part of your existence, because **simply being thankful can work miracles in your life**. People who are grateful on a regular basis:

- Are less bothered by aches and pains

- Have a stronger immune system

- Have lower blood pressure

- Exercise more and take better care of their health

- Sleep longer and feel more refreshed upon waking

- Report higher levels of positive emotions

- Feel more alert, alive, and awake

- Experience more joy and pleasure

- Have increased optimism and happiness

- Act more helpful, generous, and compassionate

- Become more forgiving

- Feel less lonely and isolated and are more outgoing

When I first heard about people practicing the art of gratitude, either in their words or with a gratitude journal, I thought it was just another fad or hype. I was already an optimistic person and was overall grateful for my life. Why did I need to add one more thing to my day? I was skeptical about whether or not it would actually work. As with anything else, I approached the gratitude concept with curiosity instead of judgement.

In Webster's dictionary, the Latin word *gratus* means "pleasing" or "thankful." At its core, gratitude is a feeling of thankfulness. I realize that we all face challenges and hard times. Gratitude doesn't mean pretending those things didn't happen. It means looking at our life in its entirety and focusing on the good.

Gratitude fills you with good feelings. When you express gratefulness for people, events, achievements, small moments, take a moment to describe the feeling in your heart. Put your hand on your chest and anchor that emotion in place.

Look outside yourself for things to be grateful for. I believe true gratitude involves being humble and acknowledging that a higher power—if you're spiritual—or other people gave us gifts, blessings, and acts of kindness. They form the basis of the goodness in our lives. Have you heard the phrase what you appreciate, appreciates? **When you focus on gratitude and being thankful, not only for the gifts but also the people or higher power behind the gifts, you will get more of that in return.**

Doing this will attract more abundance in your life with your health, love, and relationships. Your body, your health, and your relationships can only be improved by honoring where they are in this moment.

Action Step:

1. Sit down in a quiet place, take a deep breath, and place your hand on your heart. Imagine your heart filling up with glowing light. Allow this energy to fill you and radiate out from within. Begin to give thanks for your life. Give thanks for anything that comes to mind. No matter how big or small, just give thanks and appreciation.

2. Next, think of three things to be grateful for on this day. Get a visual picture in your mind. Maybe your teenager said, "*I love you mom*", or a friend texted to say she was thinking of you, or the warm day recharged you when you walked outside. Just let the images flow in and observe how you are feeling. Don't overthink it.

3. Finally, visualize the people that you are grateful for and express thanks for each of them. Think of specific gifts—emotional, physical, and spiritual—these loved ones bring to your life.

Get Quiet With Yourself

Meditation—it seems to be a buzzword right now. However, it's been around for thousands of years and is a worthwhile practice that can restore peace and quiet in your life. I used to think meditation was for "those" people. You know, the ones who did yoga every day and walked around smiling. However, I went to a retreat led by Dr. Joe Dispenza and it completely changed the way that I looked at meditation. He presented the scientific side of why meditation is not only good to help you relax and reset your current state, but also how it helps to change your *future* state.

Change can't happen by just thought alone. If this were true then we would all attain our goals. Change happens when we use all of our senses and appreciate our present state so we can visualize our future state. We then bring positive feelings to that future, and our mind and body are both on board. Just as I discussed about emotional fitness, training your mind to anticipate a bright future helps you create one.

If the idea of meditation intrigues you, I highly recommend Dr. Joe's book, *Breaking The Habit of Being Yourself*. If you spend a lot of time in your car, get the audio book. This book is not about positive thinking. It's about changing how you think, act, and feel to create a new personal reality. He doesn't just explain why you should meditate, he actually shows you how with very simple steps. He also has some amazing guided meditations that you can download or purchase. If you really want to elevate your life, go to one of his live events. Check out this YouTube video for a brief overview of his book: https://www.youtube.com/watch?v=6lbnrRqBjgE

Your thoughts have more of an impact on your life than you realize. When you wake up and dread work or complain about the early hour, you set up a pattern of negativity. If you wake up excited to start your day and move closer to your future, then you are setting yourself on a positive, productive path. If you truly want to make a change and have a different future, your thoughts have to be greater than your environment.

The best way to change your thoughts is to make time to be alone. Note I didn't say find time. *Make* time. Part of self-nourishment is making yourself a priority. We spend hours at work and come home to a family that wants more of our time. We're often already frazzled from the craziness at work and we can reach a breaking point with one more demand on our time. That's why it's vital to take a few minutes to be alone with your thoughts.

Meditation gives you the opportunity to be alone with your thoughts. It doesn't have to be anything formal or intensive. **Think of it as an opportunity to do something for yourself so you can reset your thoughts and your path for the rest of the day.** Here are a couple of short meditation techniques to get you started:

1. **Deep Breathing:** Breathing is the heart of meditation. Instead of trying to clear your mind, focus on your breaths. Remember the 5-5-7 breathing technique that was

taught in Chapter 7? Use that technique or your favorite method, or you can download an app called Breathe. It will send you text reminders during the day to breathe and focus. Choose what works for you and let your thoughts flow in and out. If your mind starts to wander, pull your focus back to your breathing. Don't judge yourself for not being able to do it "right". There is no right way. Just relax and breathe. You can do this for as little as one minute or as long as ten minutes. You can do this in your car before you leave for work, or for a minute before you head into the house at the end of the day. This is a great way to reset your nervous system by bringing you back to the present, easing the stress of the past, and preparing you for the future.

2. **Download a Meditation App:** There are so many wonderful apps out there. Some have music while others have chanting or simple breathing. One of my favorites is Simple Habit Meditation - Guided Mindfulness (featured on *Shark Tank* in October 2017). It's an app for busy people and only takes five minutes a day. They have guided meditations for specific life situations such as anxiety, depression, insomnia, etc. The app has a daily reminder to help you make this a habit. I recommend doing this either

first thing in the morning or just before you go to bed. Another great app is Calm, which has music to help you relax, sleep, or just to focus. Experiment with what works for you.

Action Step: Commit to taking five minutes a day for self-nourishment and to meditate. Approach this exercise with love and be kind to yourself. This is not one more thing for your to-do list. This is vital self-care, so that you can be your best for yourself and for others.

Chapter Ten
Ride the Healthy Highway

Congratulations! Now that you've completed this book you have invested time in yourself. You have tried a few new techniques and, because of that, you are well on your way to loving yourself to a healthy life. Think back to when you first started reading this book. What were your challenges, your goals, and your dreams? Since finishing this book, what obstacles have you overcome, how do you feel and think differently? What are some of your new goals?

If you've read this far, then you've learned that if you want to make a change and achieve extraordinary results and fulfillment in your health, you need to become laser focused on what it is you really want. Then you need to create a crystal-clear vision of where you want to go. Note, I didn't say a *plan*. I said *vision*. Having a strong image of where you want to be, engaging all of your senses so you can feel the experience and consistently visualizing it immediately changes your behavior. In turn, this will give you the momentum you need to take small actions daily. Each action leads to one big result after another, and eventually a healthy life becomes a habit.

This book is only the beginning; this is a lifestyle that will continue to unfold. I recommend you choose to implement more of these techniques and find other mindful methods to continue along the pathway for optimal health and well-being. Keep in mind that your needs will change as time progresses, and you will need to listen to your body so you can adjust your plan. What worked for you last year may no longer work this year. So keep listening to your body. It has the answers.

Acknowledge Yourself

Don't forget to acknowledge and celebrate yourself for doing such a great job. Give yourself a pat on the back and celebrate like your favorite team won the championship. Wherever you are on your journey, it's important to acknowledge and celebrate along the way. This strengthens your emotional fitness and keeps you focused on positive outcomes. As humans, we want to experience more joy, so give yourself permission to celebrate the small steps along the way.

Even after all this, you may still have a beginner's mindset. It may be too overwhelming or seem too difficult in the abstract. **Do your best to leave your criticism at the door, and adopt at least one technique that will become a *must do* versus a *should do*.** You don't have to do everything in this book nor do you have to do any of it perfectly. Think of it like taking a test drive. Pay attention to how you feel and how your energy changes. Take ten to fifteen minutes a day to tune into yourself.

As time goes by, you will find that you start naturally putting yourself first without feeling selfish. You will be healthier, more active, and more loving. You will feel joyful, peaceful, and happier. You will struggle less and live in the solution. You will be at peace in the present, whether that present is work or home or the gym. You will recognize your feelings, let go of old stories, and work through difficult times more simply.

"It is confidence in our bodies, minds, and spirits that allows us to keep looking for new adventures, new directions to grow in, and new lessons to learn-—which is what life is all about."
- Oprah Winfrey

What's the worst that can happen? This works? You find out that loving yourself was the missing link? That combining support and accountability is what you needed to live a beautiful life?

Take a deep breath and imagine the life you truly desire. Visualize that the old way of doing things like depriving, binging, negative self-talk, or skipping workouts is in the past and that you now have a plan in place and accountability to make a smooth transition to your new habits. To a new life. A new you. A new, lasting joy.

Action Step: Ask yourself these questions as you continue on your journey:

1. Am I being nourished?

2. Am I applying any of the techniques presented in this book?

3. Which ones make me energized and which ones are draining?

4. Am I committing time for myself?

5. Am I holding back or giving this my all?

6. Can I shift any of my beliefs and let go of my old story so I can embrace my desires?

7. Am I looking inward or outward to change?

8. In what ways am I celebrating my accomplishments?

9. Am I putting myself first?

10. Am I allowing myself to continue even when I mess up or am not perfect?

Embrace the New You

Sometimes we think that dreaming about more is selfish and that wanting more betrays our current reality or does a disservice to our families. I want to invite you to do both. I propose that you can love and appreciate your current reality as well as want more abundance in your life. You can only do that by releasing the past and embracing the new you.

Dissatisfaction and discouragement don't come from the absence of things, but rather from the absence of vision and the belief that you can do it. If you have an emotionally charged why and love yourself enough to give yourself permission to go after that why, you will change your life.

I say this because I have embodied this principle and witnessed it in my life and in so many others'. I started on this journey as a stressed-out career woman who was dissatisfied with her job and out of tune with both her own body and her daughter's health. To be honest, my relationship with my daughter was not as close as I desired. Only six years later, I am living my passion as an entrepreneur with a thriving health coaching business that gives me the blessing of witnessing transformations every day. I have a beautiful, healthy sixteen-year-old daughter, and our relationship is so close that we call each other best friends. And now, I'm a published author. I feel so blessed and yet

I know this is just the beginning. I know that by visualizing more I will be able to inspire others to say yes to living a beautiful life, and I will be able to contribute more to my community and to the world.

Let me ask you, what might you have to let go of in order to let yourself dream bigger and say *Yes* to yourself?

Let's take a few steps to release the past and design your new future:

Step 1. *In relation to your relationships, business/ professional aspirations, finances, health, spirituality, social, and community outreach, ask yourself the following questions:*

- Where have you improved the most?

- Where are you stuck or lacking?

- Where are you committed to going?

- Are you being stretched and challenging yourself?

- Who is your accountability partner to support and challenge yourself?

- What are your new goals and desires?

- What are you going to do to celebrate your progress?

Step 2: *Write a letter*:

- Address it: Dear (insert past year)

- Start with the new and good things that you have accomplished in all areas of your life—relationships, business/professional, finances, health, spirituality, social, and community outreach.

- Then list all of the challenges or areas that you felt stuck or were unable to accomplish.

- End the letter with a letting go statement such as: "I'm choosing to let go of _____. I'm choosing to not _____. And "I'm choosing to actively participate in my life in a fulfilling way for _____ (fill in the next year). Hello _____! (fill in the next year)

Step 3: *Write another letter*:

- Address it: Dear (current year), What I want for the New Year is:

- List all of the things that you want to accomplish in all areas of your life— relationships, business/professional, finances, health, spirituality, social, and community outreach.

- Take the letter and put it in an envelope with a stamp and address it to yourself.

- When you receive the letter in the mail, DO NOT OPEN IT!

- Put the envelope in a box and wrap it with pretty paper. Make it beautiful!

- Place it in a visible place, on your desk, kitchen, etc., where you can see it every day and be reminded of your intentions.

Step 4: On Christmas of the following year open it up and acknowledge and celebrate all of the gifts you have given yourself. Don't be critical or disappointed if you haven't accomplished them all. The important thing is to celebrate your progress. If you don't celebrate Christmas or want to do it right now, simply pick a day that is one year in the future.

This is such a fun activity and I invite you to share it with your friends and family. It's one of my favorite traditions and I hope that you will find the same in doing this.

Life is Love and Love is Life. Simple as that. We can choose to make all of this complex by overanalyzing things, people, places, events, or we can choose to let go of attachments and, as the Beatles say, *Let it be*. Choosing the latter will let love flow sweetly and freely.

Have you heard the phrase where your focus goes energy flows? This means **you need to focus on**

what you want, not on what you don't. Most people say they want to change but then talk about or think about only the things they don't like. What happens then? They don't make any changes. They stay stuck in the same rut. It's vital that you keep refocusing your lens on what you truly want. When you get sidetracked, bring your vision back around to what's possible.

In this book, we have covered a lot of information I know that can be overwhelming, so I've summarized everything I talked about into three steps:

1. Be Present and Curious

2. Nourish Your Mind, Body, Emotions

3. Love Yourself, Contribute, Be Grateful

The methods and techniques that I have presented all encompass these three steps. One of the keys to lasting habit change is to find the right system or method that works for you. I laid out many steps in this book and I encourage you to take each one for a test drive before discounting any of them outright.

To achieve lasting habit change you don't need to use force, deprivation, self-criticism, willpower, or exterior motivators. Simply keep your focus on why you want to change, then take a moment to slow down, step back and look at your behaviors, beliefs, and stories with a curious mind. From there, you can make gradual changes in your language, thoughts, and actions until they align with your values. Sometimes you have to slow down to speed up.

The most valuable part of this equation is you. **You need to believe in yourself before any of this takes hold.** When you start to value yourself and work on your inner world, your outer world will come into alignment. You will make different choices without even having to think about what you are doing.

Having the right method or system is only one piece of the puzzle. Many of my clients fear they will sabotage their success, or that what they are doing is not sustainable. With our hectic lives, it is really difficult to do everything on our own. You've heard the phrase *it takes a village to raise a child*. It takes a village to maintain our health. Women, especially, need support. When we try to do everything ourselves, we end up burning out and giving up on ourselves.

Believe it or not, I have a coach and a business mentor for myself. My clients often ask me why I need a coach if I am a coach. I have one because I believe in the power of coaching and accountability. It's not just about someone supporting you, it's about someone holding the space for a bigger vision for you and stretching you to achieve it.

So, the second key component for creating lasting habit change is to find the right support and accountability. You can hire a coach, mentor, or even find a friend to support you and to be your accountability partner. Be selective with who you choose. You want to find someone who will stretch you so that you will grow. Someone who can cheer you on when you start to lose focus or get frustrated and someone who can give you a little kick in the rear when you start to live in your excuses and not the solution.

If you only find someone for support you will stay in a comfortable state. You may make some progress but it will be so slow that it will not be fulfilling and you'll give up. While support sounds nice, without the stretch of accountability you will not be setting yourself up for success. Most of us know what to do, we just don't always do it. **What's standing between you knowing what to do and actually doing it is accountability.**

Action Step: The last action step is one that I am going to leave up to you. I am trusting that I have empowered you with the tools to assist you in taking the next step forward to being an advocate for your own health. If my work resonated with you and you are clearly committed to creating a better relationship with your health and life and believe that my work can be of service to this goal, then I invite you to schedule a fifteen-minute Body-Life breakthrough session by phone to see if we are a good fit.

If you're interested, go to this link for my online scheduler: https://www.stacysolie.com/services. I would love to partner with you to release the past and move forward into the body and life of your dreams. Whether you decide to connect with me or look for other options, I encourage you to find someone who will be your accountability partner. Set some intentions and find someone who loves you enough to encourage you to stretch toward your dreams.

My intention has been to inspire you with knowledge and techniques to remind yourself of the power that lies within you. At the end of all of this, I hope that you have a greater belief of the truly magnificent being that you truly are.

I believe everyone can learn to behave differently and everyone can learn to create a beautiful state. Everyone can love themselves healthy, and love themselves for the rest of their lives. Believe in that, and believe in yourself, because I believe in you! You are worth it!

Appendix A

Mindset Makeover

Seven Areas to Reshape Your Health and Keep it Super Simple

These seven areas represent one way of evaluating a healthy life. The exercise measures your levels of satisfaction in the present moment. It is not a picture of how it has been in the past or what you want it to be in the future. It is a snapshot taken in the moment. The emphasis is on your level of satisfaction in each area.

Rate your level of satisfaction in all seven areas of your life. Zero means not satisfied and ten means highly satisfied. Remember, this is not about getting tens! It's about a smoother ride. The goal is not to criticize yourself or be disappointed. The goal is for you to step back from your current situation so you can get a clear visual of any imbalances. That gives you a starting point where you may wish to spend more time and energy to create balance and joy and improve your overall health.

Circle your level of satisfaction:

1. Love/relationships:

1   2   3   4   5   6   7   8   9   10

2. Business/Career:

1   2   3   4   5   6   7   8   9   10

3. Movement/Exercise:

1   2   3   4   5   6   7   8   9   10

4. Nourishment/Food:

1   2   3   4   5   6   7   8   9   10

5. Self-Care/Gratitude:

1   2   3   4   5   6   7   8   9   10

6. Fun/Social:

1   2   3   4   5   6   7   8   9   10

7. Spirituality:

1   2   3   4   5   6   7   8   9   10

I encourage you to reach out for support so you can hold yourself accountable to ensure your success. Remember, you are worth it and so is your health!

Appendix B

Eating Mindfully Chart

Day	Time	Feeling	Satiated	Noticed
SAMPLE				
Day One	6	Not Sure	Not Sure	I eat faster than I thought
Day Two	11	Anxious	I think so	I don't really know if this will work for me
Day Three	16	Easier	I think 15	This is getting easier

Day	Time	Feeling	Satiated	Noticed
<u>YOUR TURN</u>				
Day One				
Day Two				
Day Three				

About the Author

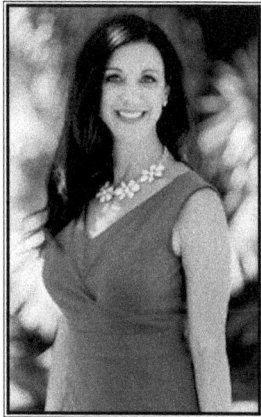

Founder of Healthy Weight Naturally, Stacy Solie is a highly sought after health coach, author and speaker based in Palm Harbor, Florida. A Board Certified Holistic Health Coach, Stacy is passionate about helping women tap into their core potential to live an energized, balanced and deeply fulfilled life while looking and feeling their best. She is trained in over one hundred dietary theories, practical lifestyle management techniques, NLP, TCM, and other innovative coaching methods. She has studied with and learned from some of the world's top health and wellness experts, including Dr. Andrew Weil, Dr. Deepak Chopra, Dr. David Katz, Dr. Walter Willett, Geneen Roth, Dr. Joe Dispenza, Jeffery Combs, Stacey Morgenstern, Carey Peters, and Tony Robbins. She is dedicated to inspiring her clients to love themselves healthy so they can stop holding back and start living the beautiful life they desire and deserve!

Connect with the Author

Facebook:
http://facebook.com/stacysoliecoaching

Instagram:
https://www.instagram.com/stacysoliecoaching/

Website:
www.stacysolie.com

Email:
Stacy@stacysolie.com